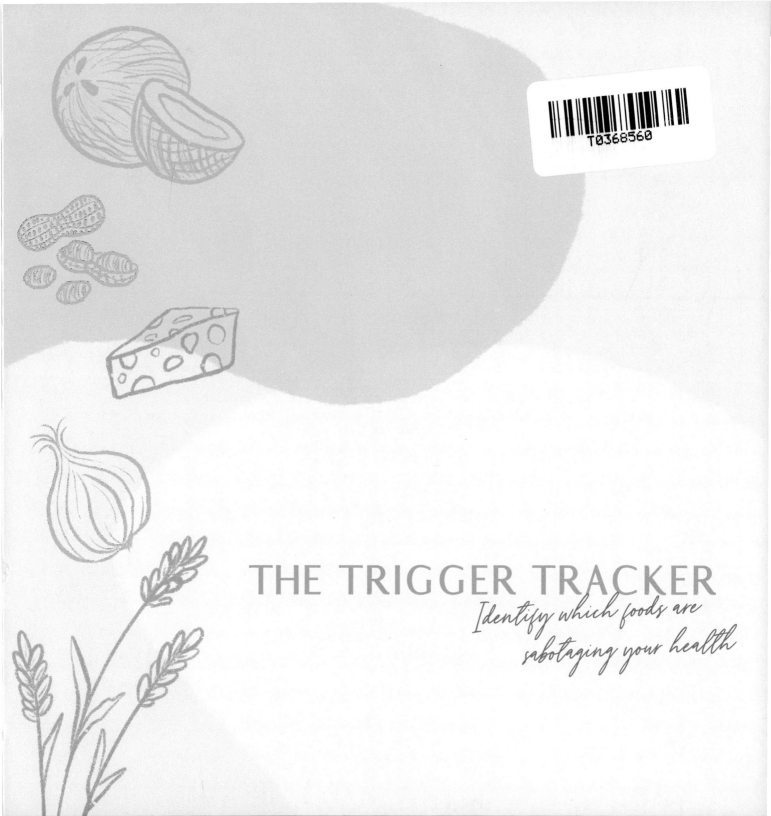

# THE TRIGGER TRACKER

*Identify which foods are*
*sabotaging your health*

AuthorHouse™
1663 Liberty Drive
Bloomington, IN 47403
www.authorhouse.com
Phone: 833-262-8899

Because of the dynamic nature of the Internet, any web addresses or links contained in this book may have changed
since publication and may no longer be valid. The views expressed in this work are solely those of the author and do
not necessarily reflect the views of the publisher, and the publisher hereby disclaims any responsibility for them.

Any people depicted in stock imagery provided by Getty Images are models,
and such images are being used for illustrative purposes only.
Certain stock imagery © Getty Images.

This book is printed on acid-free paper.

ISBN: 978-1-6655-5025-3 (sc)
ISBN: 978-1-6655-5024-6 (e)

Library of Congress Control Number: 2022901219

Print information available on the last page.

Published by AuthorHouse  01/21/2022

authorHOUSE

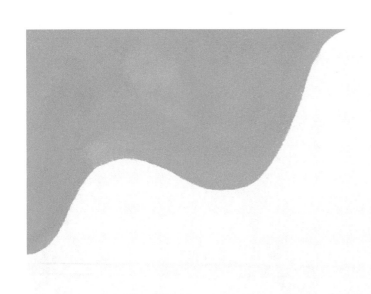

THIS TRIGGER TRACKER BELONGS TO:

................................................................................................

STARTING ON ......../......../..................

MY BIGGEST HEALTH CONCERNS ARE:

......................................................................................................................................
......................................................................................................................................
......................................................................................................................................
......................................................................................................................................
......................................................................................................................................

MY HEALTH GOALS ARE:

......................................................................................................................................
......................................................................................................................................
......................................................................................................................................
......................................................................................................................................
......................................................................................................................................

ANYTHING ELSE I WANT TO SHARE:

......................................................................................................................................
......................................................................................................................................
......................................................................................................................................
......................................................................................................................................
......................................................................................................................................
......................................................................................................................................
......................................................................................................................................

TO HELP YOU GET CRYSTAL CLEAR ON WHAT YOU WANT, VISIT:
*WWW.THETRIGGERTRACKERJOURNAL.COM/BONUSES*

# FOOD TRACKING.
# MADE EASY.

You want to lose weight to feel good. And, if you're like most people, you're probably willing to put yourself through hell to get there.

But what if I told you you didn't have to do that? What if I told you there is another way to drop weight? To feel good?

If you're skeptical, I get it. After all, we've been conditioned to believe that if we want to drop weight, burn fat, or get healthy - we have to endure pain.

But let me ask you something: If the end goal of weight loss is to feel good, doesn't it make sense that you have to feel good during the process?

Of course it does.

I mean, you don't get freedom through shackles, so why would you try to feel good by feeling bad first?

It just doesn't make sense. But it's what we've been taught to do.

Which is why so many of us have failed at keeping the weight off. Because we've bought into the lie that weight loss comes before feeling good.

But it doesn't. Real weight loss, the kind that keeps the pounds from coming back, comes from feeling good first.

Which is why I'm so glad you're here. Because if you picked up The Trigger Tracker—you're looking for a real solution. You're looking for sustainable weight loss.

And I like that about you. Which is why I'm going to tell you the secret the diet industry has been keeping from you: sustainable weight loss is a byproduct of feeling good.

That's right. To drop weight sustainably you have to feel good during the weight loss process. Hence why this food journal isn't about tracking calories or macros and, instead, is all about tracking which foods make you feel good and which ones don't.

Because you have to eliminate foods that don't make you feel good to feel good. Because when you eat foods that don't feel so good, you cause unnecessary and excess inflammation in your system. And that works against your goals.

Also, if left unchecked, inflammation in your system leads to obesity, metabolic diseases like type 2 diabetes, and gut issues like IBS. And you don't want that.

Which is why you're here. Because you kinda know that something you're eating isn't doing you any favors. And you've probably come to the conclusion that what you were doing to drop weight isn't working either. And you're probably over your stomach hurting all the time and the bloating that comes with it.

Exactly—which, again, is why I'm so glad you're here. Because The Trigger Tracker was designed for someone like you. Someone who is convinced there is another way to do this whole weight loss thing. And someone who is ready to just feel good.

So, welcome to your solution, friend. Because this tracker—well, it's going to show you how to do just that.

With love,

*Erica*

Erica

# GETTING THE MOST

## STEP 1:
Pick an elimination diet to execute over 21 days.

**Basic Elimination Diet***
- No Dairy
- No Eggs
- No Gluten
- No Soy

**Liver-based Elimination Diet***
- No Added Sugar (artificial or real)
- No Alcohol
- No Caffeine
- No Dairy
- No Gluten
- No Soy

**Your Choice**
- Your Own Elimination Diet
- Whole30
- Doctor-Recommended Elimination Diet
- Other Elimination Diet (e.g. The Plan, nightshade elimination)

**Autoimmune Elimination Diet****
- No Artificial Sweeteners, Stevia and Xylitol
- No Chocolate (including cacao)
- No Dairy
- No Eggs
- No Beans Legumes (including peanuts)
- No Grains (whole or processed)
- No Processed Foods
- No Nightshades
- No Nuts or Seeds (including herb seeds—mustard seeds, coriander seeds, fennel, fenugreek)
- No Tapioca
- No Vegetable, Canola, Cottonseed or Soybean-based Oil

\* Recommended for someone living with an autoimmune condition
\* For elimination-diet friendly recipes and meal plans, visit **www.thetriggertrackerjournal.com/recipes**

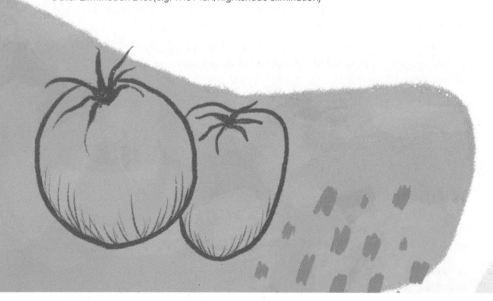

# OUT OF YOUR JOURNAL

### STEP 2:

Track all meals, being sure to list the food you ate, time of day you ate it, and any negative feelings following the food's consumption.

### STEP 3:

On Day 22, reintroduce one food item you eliminated back into your diet over a period of three days to see if/how it affects your body.

### STEP 4:

On Day 25, reintroduce another food item you eliminated back into your diet over a period of three days to see if/how it affects your body.

### STEP 5:

Continue to reintroduce eliminated foods back into your diet every three days to determine if they trigger you, i.e. if they are causing unnecessary inflammation in your body. Depending on the protocol you choose, the Trigger Tracker Process will take:

- **Basic Elimination Diet:**
  33 days (with reintroductions on Day 22, 25, 28, 31...)

- **Liver-based Elimination Diet:**
  39 days (with reintroductions on Day 22, 25, 28, 31...)

- **Autoimmune Elimination Diet:**
  54 days (with reintroductions on Day 22, 25, 28, 31...)

- **Your Choice:** 21 days + (3 x # of items you will add back in) days

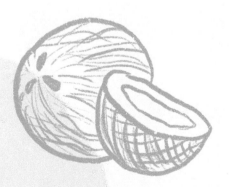

## THINGS NOT TO DO:

Track calories

Count macros

Skip the journal prompts

Beat yourself up for not knowing better, for not starting sooner, and/ or not being at the weight you want to be at yet.

........ / ........ / ............

## SLEEP:

🌙 ............ HOURS OF SLEEP LAST NIGHT

## EXERCISE:

BIKE　　SWIM　　YOGA

WALK/HIKE　　WEIGHTS　　CARDIO

OTHER ACTIVITY:

............................................

TOTAL TIME
EXERCISING: ........................

## WATER INTAKE:

8 oz　8 oz　8 oz　8 oz　8 oz

8 oz　8 oz　8 oz　8 oz　8 oz

## ENERGY:

0　2　4　6　8　10

⊖ · · · · · · · · · ⊕

## STRESS:

0　2　4　6　8　10

❄ · · · · · · · · · 🔥

**BREAKFAST**

____:____ AM/PM

FOODS:

HOW DO I FEEL?

**LUNCH**

____:____ AM/PM

FOODS:

HOW DO I FEEL?

**DINNER**

____:____ AM/PM

FOODS:

HOW DO I FEEL?

**SNACKS**

____:____ AM/PM

FOODS:

HOW DO I FEEL?

## MOOD:

EXPLAIN WHY:

## NOTES:

......................................................
......................................................
......................................................
......................................................
......................................................

......... / ......... / .............

## SLEEP:

🌙 ............. HOURS OF SLEEP LAST NIGHT

## EXERCISE:

BIKE    SWIM    YOGA

WALK/HIKE    WEIGHTS    CARDIO

OTHER ACTIVITY:

......................................

TOTAL TIME EXERCISING: .................

## WATER INTAKE:

8 oz   8 oz   8 oz   8 oz   8 oz

8 oz   8 oz   8 oz   8 oz   8 oz

## ENERGY:

| 0 | 2 | 4 | 6 | 8 | 10 |

⊖ · ı · ı · ı · ı · ⊕

## STRESS:

| 0 | 2 | 4 | 6 | 8 | 10 |

❄ · ı · ı · ı · ı · 🔥

**BREAKFAST**   ____:____ AM/PM   FOODS:     HOW DO I FEEL?

**LUNCH**   ____:____ AM/PM   FOODS:     HOW DO I FEEL?

**DINNER**   ____:____ AM/PM   FOODS:     HOW DO I FEEL?

**SNACKS**   ____:____ AM/PM   FOODS:     HOW DO I FEEL?

## MOOD:

EXPLAIN WHY:

## NOTES:

........................................................
........................................................
........................................................
........................................................
........................................................

......... /......... /.............

## SLEEP:

................ HOURS OF SLEEP LAST NIGHT

## EXERCISE:

BIKE   SWIM   YOGA

WALK/HIKE   WEIGHTS   CARDIO

OTHER ACTIVITY:

.........................................

TOTAL TIME
EXERCISING:

## WATER INTAKE:

8 oz  8 oz  8 oz  8 oz  8 oz

8 oz  8 oz  8 oz  8 oz  8 oz

## ENERGY:

0   2   4   6   8   10

⊖ · ' ' ' ' ' ' · ⊕

## STRESS:

0   2   4   6   8   10

❋ · ' ' ' ' ' ' · 🔥

**BREAKFAST**

____:____AM/PM
FOODS:

HOW DO I FEEL?

**LUNCH**

____:____AM/PM
FOODS:

HOW DO I FEEL?

**DINNER**

____:____AM/PM
FOODS:

HOW DO I FEEL?

**SNACKS**

____:____AM/PM
FOODS:

HOW DO I FEEL?

## MOOD:

EXPLAIN WHY:

## NOTES:

..................................................
..................................................
..................................................
..................................................
..................................................

........../........../...............

## SLEEP:

🌙 ............... HOURS OF SLEEP LAST NIGHT

## EXERCISE:

BIKE          SWIM          YOGA

WALK/HIKE     WEIGHTS       CARDIO

OTHER ACTIVITY:

...............................................

TOTAL TIME
EXERCISING: 

## WATER INTAKE:

8 oz    8 oz    8 oz    8 oz    8 oz

8 oz    8 oz    8 oz    8 oz    8 oz

## ENERGY:

| 0 | 2 | 4 | 6 | 8 | 10 |
|---|---|---|---|---|---|
| − | · | · | · | · | + |

## STRESS:

| 0 | 2 | 4 | 6 | 8 | 10 |
|---|---|---|---|---|---|
| ❄ | · | · | · | · | 🔥 |

**BREAKFAST**

____:____AM/PM
FOODS:

HOW DO I FEEL?

**LUNCH**

____:____AM/PM
FOODS:

HOW DO I FEEL?

**DINNER**

____:____AM/PM
FOODS:

HOW DO I FEEL?

**SNACKS**

____:____AM/PM
FOODS:

HOW DO I FEEL?

## MOOD:

EXPLAIN WHY:

## NOTES:

..........................................................
..........................................................
..........................................................
..........................................................
..........................................................

**WHAT DO I NEED TO DO
TO ENSURE I CONTINUE TO FOLLOW
THROUGH ON THIS ELIMINATION DIET?**

.................................................................................................
.................................................................................................
.................................................................................................
.................................................................................................
.................................................................................................
.................................................................................................
.................................................................................................
.................................................................................................
.................................................................................................
.................................................................................................
.................................................................................................
.................................................................................................

.........../........../..............

## SLEEP:

🌙 ............ HOURS OF SLEEP LAST NIGHT

## EXERCISE:

🚲
BIKE

🏊
SWIM

🧘
YOGA

👟
WALK/HIKE

🏋️
WEIGHTS

🏃
CARDIO

❤️
OTHER ACTIVITY:

.......................................

⏱️ TOTAL TIME EXERCISING:

## WATER INTAKE:

8 oz   8 oz   8 oz   8 oz   8 oz

8 oz   8 oz   8 oz   8 oz   8 oz

## ENERGY:

| 0 | 2 | 4 | 6 | 8 | 10 |
|---|---|---|---|---|---|

⊖ · · ı · ı · ı · ⊕

## STRESS:

| 0 | 2 | 4 | 6 | 8 | 10 |
|---|---|---|---|---|---|

❄️ · · ı · ı · ı · 🔥

### BREAKFAST
_____:_____ AM/PM
FOODS:

HOW DO I FEEL?

### LUNCH
_____:_____ AM/PM
FOODS:

HOW DO I FEEL?

### DINNER
_____:_____ AM/PM
FOODS:

HOW DO I FEEL?

### SNACKS
_____:_____ AM/PM
FOODS:

HOW DO I FEEL?

## MOOD:

EXPLAIN WHY:

## NOTES:

....................................................

....................................................

....................................................

....................................................

....................................................

.......... / ......... / .............

## SLEEP:

.............. HOURS OF SLEEP LAST NIGHT

## EXERCISE:

BIKE          SWIM          YOGA

WALK/HIKE     WEIGHTS       CARDIO

OTHER ACTIVITY:

.......................................................

TOTAL TIME
EXERCISING:

## WATER INTAKE:

8 oz    8 oz    8 oz    8 oz    8 oz

8 oz    8 oz    8 oz    8 oz    8 oz

## ENERGY:

0    2    4    6    8    10

⊖                            ⊕

## STRESS:

0    2    4    6    8    10

❋                            ◑

**BREAKFAST**

_____:_____ AM/PM

FOODS:

HOW DO I FEEL?

**LUNCH**

_____:_____ AM/PM

FOODS:

HOW DO I FEEL?

**DINNER**

_____:_____ AM/PM

FOODS:

HOW DO I FEEL?

**SNACKS**

_____:_____ AM/PM

FOODS:

HOW DO I FEEL?

## MOOD:

EXPLAIN WHY:

## NOTES:

.........................................................................
.........................................................................
.........................................................................
.........................................................................
.........................................................................

......... / ......... / .............

## SLEEP:

☾ ............. HOURS OF SLEEP LAST NIGHT

## EXERCISE:

🚲 BIKE

🏊 SWIM

🧘 YOGA

👟 WALK/HIKE

🏋 WEIGHTS

🏃 CARDIO

💗 OTHER ACTIVITY:

.........................................

⏱ TOTAL TIME EXERCISING:

## WATER INTAKE:

8 oz · 8 oz · 8 oz · 8 oz · 8 oz

8 oz · 8 oz · 8 oz · 8 oz · 8 oz

## ENERGY:

| 0 | 2 | 4 | 6 | 8 | 10 |
|---|---|---|---|---|---|

⊖ · · · · · · · · · ⊕

## STRESS:

| 0 | 2 | 4 | 6 | 8 | 10 |
|---|---|---|---|---|---|

❄ · · · · · · · · · 🔥

**BREAKFAST**

_____:_____ AM/PM

FOODS:

HOW DO I FEEL?

**LUNCH**

_____:_____ AM/PM

FOODS:

HOW DO I FEEL?

**DINNER**

_____:_____ AM/PM

FOODS:

HOW DO I FEEL?

**SNACKS**

_____:_____ AM/PM

FOODS:

HOW DO I FEEL?

## MOOD:

😖 😕 😐 🙂 😀

EXPLAIN WHY:

## NOTES:

........................................................
........................................................
........................................................
........................................................
........................................................

HOW DO I FEEL RIGHT NOW?

........................................................................................................

........................................................................................................

........................................................................................................

........................................................................................................

........................................................................................................

WHAT DO I NEED TO SHIFT TO FEEL EVEN BETTER THAN I DO NOW?

........................................................................................................

........................................................................................................

........................................................................................................

........................................................................................................

........................................................................................................

HOW CAN I MAKE THOSE SHIFTS?

........................................................................................................

........................................................................................................

........................................................................................................

........................................................................................................

........................................................................................................

WHAT HAS TO CHANGE IN MY DAY-TO-DAY LIFE
TO  INCORPORATE THESE SHIFTS?

........................................................................................................

........................................................................................................

........................................................................................................

........................................................................................................

........................................................................................................

......... / ......... / ...............

## SLEEP:

🌙 ............ HOURS OF SLEEP LAST NIGHT

## EXERCISE:

BIKE

SWIM

YOGA

WALK/HIKE

WEIGHTS

CARDIO

OTHER ACTIVITY:

.............................................

TOTAL TIME
EXERCISING:

## WATER INTAKE:

8 oz  8 oz  8 oz  8 oz  8 oz

8 oz  8 oz  8 oz  8 oz  8 oz

## ENERGY:

| 0 | 2 | 4 | 6 | 8 | 10 |
|---|---|---|---|---|----|

⊖ . . ı . ı . ı . ⊕

## STRESS:

| 0 | 2 | 4 | 6 | 8 | 10 |
|---|---|---|---|---|----|

❄ . . ı . ı . ı . 🔥

**BREAKFAST**
____:____ AM/PM
FOODS:

HOW DO I FEEL?

**LUNCH**
____:____ AM/PM
FOODS:

HOW DO I FEEL?

**DINNER**
____:____ AM/PM
FOODS:

HOW DO I FEEL?

**SNACKS**
____:____ AM/PM
FOODS:

HOW DO I FEEL?

## MOOD:

😠 😟 😐 🙂 😄

EXPLAIN WHY:

## NOTES:

.........................................................
.........................................................
.........................................................
.........................................................
.........................................................

........../........../..............

## SLEEP:

(  .............. HOURS OF SLEEP LAST NIGHT

## EXERCISE:

BIKE          SWIM          YOGA

WALK/HIKE     WEIGHTS       CARDIO

OTHER ACTIVITY:

.................................................

TOTAL TIME
EXERCISING: ..............................

## WATER INTAKE:

8 oz    8 oz    8 oz    8 oz    8 oz

8 oz    8 oz    8 oz    8 oz    8 oz

## ENERGY:

0    2    4    6    8    10

⊖    .    .    .    .    .    .    .    ⊕

## STRESS:

0    2    4    6    8    10

❄    .    .    .    .    .    .    .    🔥

**BREAKFAST**

_____:_____ AM/PM

FOODS:

HOW DO I FEEL?

**LUNCH**

_____:_____ AM/PM

FOODS:

HOW DO I FEEL?

**DINNER**

_____:_____ AM/PM

FOODS:

HOW DO I FEEL?

**SNACKS**

_____:_____ AM/PM

FOODS:

HOW DO I FEEL?

## MOOD:

EXPLAIN WHY:

## NOTES:

.............................................................

.............................................................

.............................................................

.............................................................

.............................................................

......... / ........ / ..............

## SLEEP:

🌙 ............... HOURS OF SLEEP LAST NIGHT

## EXERCISE:

BIKE          SWIM          YOGA

WALK/HIKE     WEIGHTS       CARDIO

OTHER ACTIVITY:

..............................................

TOTAL TIME
EXERCISING:

## WATER INTAKE:

8 oz   8 oz   8 oz   8 oz   8 oz

8 oz   8 oz   8 oz   8 oz   8 oz

## ENERGY:

| 0 | 2 | 4 | 6 | 8 | 10 |
|---|---|---|---|---|----|

⊖ · · | · | · | · · ⊕

## STRESS:

| 0 | 2 | 4 | 6 | 8 | 10 |
|---|---|---|---|---|----|

❄ · · | · | · | · · 🔥

---

**BREAKFAST** ____:____ AM/PM
FOODS:

HOW DO I FEEL?

**LUNCH** ____:____ AM/PM
FOODS:

HOW DO I FEEL?

**DINNER** ____:____ AM/PM
FOODS:

HOW DO I FEEL?

**SNACKS** ____:____ AM/PM
FOODS:

HOW DO I FEEL?

## MOOD:

EXPLAIN WHY:

## NOTES:

..........................................................................
..........................................................................
..........................................................................
..........................................................................
..........................................................................

........ / ........ / ..............

## SLEEP:

🌙 ............. HOURS OF SLEEP LAST NIGHT

## EXERCISE:

BIKE     SWIM     YOGA

WALK/HIKE    WEIGHTS    CARDIO

OTHER ACTIVITY:

..................................................

TOTAL TIME
EXERCISING:

## WATER INTAKE:

8 oz   8 oz   8 oz   8 oz   8 oz

8 oz   8 oz   8 oz   8 oz   8 oz

## ENERGY:

| 0 | 2 | 4 | 6 | 8 | 10 |
|---|---|---|---|---|----|

⊖   ·   '   '   '   '   ·   ⊕

## STRESS:

| 0 | 2 | 4 | 6 | 8 | 10 |
|---|---|---|---|---|----|

❄   ·   '   '   '   '   ·   🔥

### BREAKFAST

_____:_____ AM/PM
FOODS:

HOW DO I FEEL?

### LUNCH

_____:_____ AM/PM
FOODS:

HOW DO I FEEL?

### DINNER

_____:_____ AM/PM
FOODS:

HOW DO I FEEL?

### SNACKS

_____:_____ AM/PM
FOODS:

HOW DO I FEEL?

## MOOD:

😖   😕   😐   🙂   😄

| | | | | |
|---|---|---|---|---|

EXPLAIN WHY:

## NOTES:

..................................................................
..................................................................
..................................................................
..................................................................
..................................................................

## HOW DOES STRESS AFFECT MY FOOD DECISIONS?

## WHAT CAN I DO ABOUT MY STRESS?

......... / ......... / .............

## SLEEP:

( .............. HOURS OF SLEEP LAST NIGHT

## EXERCISE:

BIKE　　SWIM　　YOGA

WALK/HIKE　WEIGHTS　CARDIO

OTHER ACTIVITY:

.................................................

TOTAL TIME
EXERCISING: .........................

## WATER INTAKE:

8 oz　8 oz　8 oz　8 oz　8 oz

8 oz　8 oz　8 oz　8 oz　8 oz

## ENERGY:

0　2　4　6　8　10

⊖ · · · · · · · · ⊕

## STRESS:

0　2　4　6　8　10

❋ · · · · · · · · 🔥

**BREAKFAST**　____:____ AM/PM　FOODS:　HOW DO I FEEL?

**LUNCH**　____:____ AM/PM　FOODS:　HOW DO I FEEL?

**DINNER**　____:____ AM/PM　FOODS:　HOW DO I FEEL?

**SNACKS**　____:____ AM/PM　FOODS:　HOW DO I FEEL?

## MOOD:

EXPLAIN WHY:

## NOTES:

...........................................................
...........................................................
...........................................................
...........................................................
...........................................................

......... /......... /...............

## SLEEP:

🌙 .............. HOURS OF SLEEP LAST NIGHT

## EXERCISE:

BIKE          SWIM          YOGA

WALK/HIKE     WEIGHTS       CARDIO

OTHER ACTIVITY:

.............................................

TOTAL TIME
EXERCISING: ...................................

## WATER INTAKE:

8 oz   8 oz   8 oz   8 oz   8 oz

8 oz   8 oz   8 oz   8 oz   8 oz

## ENERGY:

| 0 | 2 | 4 | 6 | 8 | 10 |
|---|---|---|---|---|----|

⊖ · · · · · · · · ⊕

## STRESS:

| 0 | 2 | 4 | 6 | 8 | 10 |
|---|---|---|---|---|----|

❄ · · · · · · · · 🔥

**BREAKFAST**

_____:_____ AM/PM
FOODS:

HOW DO I FEEL?

**LUNCH**

_____:_____ AM/PM
FOODS:

HOW DO I FEEL?

**DINNER**

_____:_____ AM/PM
FOODS:

HOW DO I FEEL?

**SNACKS**

_____:_____ AM/PM
FOODS:

HOW DO I FEEL?

## MOOD:

EXPLAIN WHY:

## NOTES:

.............................................................

.............................................................

.............................................................

.............................................................

.............................................................

......... / ......... / .............

## SLEEP:

.............. HOURS OF SLEEP LAST NIGHT

## EXERCISE:

BIKE     SWIM     YOGA

WALK/HIKE     WEIGHTS     CARDIO

OTHER ACTIVITY:

......................................

TOTAL TIME
EXERCISING: ...............................

## WATER INTAKE:

8 oz   8 oz   8 oz   8 oz   8 oz

8 oz   8 oz   8 oz   8 oz   8 oz

## ENERGY:

0   2   4   6   8   10

⊖   ⊕

## STRESS:

0   2   4   6   8   10

**BREAKFAST**

____:____AM/PM

FOODS:

HOW DO I FEEL?

**LUNCH**

____:____AM/PM

FOODS:

HOW DO I FEEL?

**DINNER**

____:____AM/PM

FOODS:

HOW DO I FEEL?

**SNACKS**

____:____AM/PM

FOODS:

HOW DO I FEEL?

## MOOD:

EXPLAIN WHY:

## NOTES:

...............................................................
...............................................................
...............................................................
...............................................................
...............................................................

WHY HAVE I BEEN EATING FOODS THAT DON'T MAKE ME FEEL GOOD?

........................................................................................
........................................................................................
........................................................................................
........................................................................................
........................................................................................
........................................................................................

HOW WAS THAT SERVING ME?

........................................................................................
........................................................................................
........................................................................................
........................................................................................
........................................................................................
........................................................................................

WHAT DO I THINK THOSE FOODS ARE DOING FOR ME?

........................................................................................
........................................................................................
........................................................................................
........................................................................................
........................................................................................
........................................................................................
........................................................................................

.........../........../.............

## SLEEP:

( ............... HOURS OF SLEEP LAST NIGHT

## EXERCISE:

BIKE SWIM YOGA

WALK/HIKE WEIGHTS CARDIO

OTHER ACTIVITY:

...............................................

TOTAL TIME
EXERCISING:

## WATER INTAKE:

8 oz 8 oz 8 oz 8 oz 8 oz

8 oz 8 oz 8 oz 8 oz 8 oz

## ENERGY:

0 2 4 6 8 10

—   +

## STRESS:

0 2 4 6 8 10

**BREAKFAST** _____:_____ AM/PM
FOODS:

HOW DO I FEEL?

**LUNCH** _____:_____ AM/PM
FOODS:

HOW DO I FEEL?

**DINNER** _____:_____ AM/PM
FOODS:

HOW DO I FEEL?

**SNACKS** _____:_____ AM/PM
FOODS:

HOW DO I FEEL?

## MOOD:

EXPLAIN WHY:

## NOTES:

...................................................
...................................................
...................................................
...................................................
...................................................

........../........../.............

## SLEEP:

🌙 ............. HOURS OF SLEEP LAST NIGHT

## EXERCISE:

🚲 BIKE     🏊 SWIM     🧘 YOGA

👟 WALK/HIKE     🏋 WEIGHTS     🏃 CARDIO

💗 OTHER ACTIVITY:

............................................

⏱ TOTAL TIME EXERCISING: ........................

## WATER INTAKE:

8 oz   8 oz   8 oz   8 oz   8 oz

8 oz   8 oz   8 oz   8 oz   8 oz

## ENERGY:

0   2   4   6   8   10

⊖    ⊕

## STRESS:

0   2   4   6   8   10

❄    🔥

**BREAKFAST**

_____:_____ AM/PM

FOODS:

HOW DO I FEEL?

**LUNCH**

_____:_____ AM/PM

FOODS:

HOW DO I FEEL?

**DINNER**

_____:_____ AM/PM

FOODS:

HOW DO I FEEL?

**SNACKS**

_____:_____ AM/PM

FOODS:

HOW DO I FEEL?

## MOOD:

EXPLAIN WHY:

## NOTES:

..................................................
..................................................
..................................................
..................................................
..................................................

........ / ........ / .............

## SLEEP:

............. HOURS OF SLEEP LAST NIGHT

## EXERCISE:

BIKE        SWIM        YOGA

WALK/HIKE   WEIGHTS     CARDIO

OTHER ACTIVITY:
....................................................

TOTAL TIME
EXERCISING: ...........................

## WATER INTAKE:

8 oz   8 oz   8 oz   8 oz   8 oz

8 oz   8 oz   8 oz   8 oz   8 oz

## ENERGY:

0    2    4    6    8    10
⊖ · · · · · · · · · ⊕

## STRESS:

0    2    4    6    8    10
❋ · · · · · · · · · 🔥

### BREAKFAST

_____:_____ AM/PM
FOODS:

HOW DO I FEEL?

### LUNCH

_____:_____ AM/PM
FOODS:

HOW DO I FEEL?

### DINNER

_____:_____ AM/PM
FOODS:

HOW DO I FEEL?

### SNACKS

_____:_____ AM/PM
FOODS:

HOW DO I FEEL?

## MOOD:

EXPLAIN WHY:

## NOTES:

..............................................................
..............................................................
..............................................................
..............................................................
..............................................................

........../......../..............

## SLEEP:

🌙 ............... HOURS OF SLEEP LAST NIGHT

## EXERCISE:

🚲 BIKE

🏊 SWIM

🧘 YOGA

👟 WALK/HIKE

🏋 WEIGHTS

🏃 CARDIO

💗 OTHER ACTIVITY:

.................................................

⏱ TOTAL TIME EXERCISING:

## WATER INTAKE:

8 oz   8 oz   8 oz   8 oz   8 oz

8 oz   8 oz   8 oz   8 oz   8 oz

## ENERGY:

| 0 | 2 | 4 | 6 | 8 | 10 |
|---|---|---|---|---|---|

⊖ · · ' · ' · ' · · ⊕

## STRESS:

| 0 | 2 | 4 | 6 | 8 | 10 |
|---|---|---|---|---|---|

❄ · · ' · ' · ' · · 🔥

**BREAKFAST**

_____:_____ AM/PM
FOODS:

HOW DO I FEEL?

**LUNCH**

_____:_____ AM/PM
FOODS:

HOW DO I FEEL?

**DINNER**

_____:_____ AM/PM
FOODS:

HOW DO I FEEL?

**SNACKS**

_____:_____ AM/PM
FOODS:

HOW DO I FEEL?

## MOOD:

😠 😕 😐 🙂 😄

EXPLAIN WHY:

## NOTES:

...........................................................
...........................................................
...........................................................
...........................................................
...........................................................

WHAT IS THE BIGGEST LESSON I'VE LEARNED SO FAR
DURING THIS ELIMINATION DIET?

......... / ........ / .............

## SLEEP:

☾ ............. HOURS OF SLEEP LAST NIGHT

## EXERCISE:

BIKE   SWIM   YOGA

WALK/HIKE   WEIGHTS   CARDIO

OTHER ACTIVITY:

..............................................

TOTAL TIME
EXERCISING:

## WATER INTAKE:

8 oz  8 oz  8 oz  8 oz  8 oz

8 oz  8 oz  8 oz  8 oz  8 oz

## ENERGY:

| 0 | 2 | 4 | 6 | 8 | 10 |
|---|---|---|---|---|----|

⊖ · · · · · · · ⊕

## STRESS:

| 0 | 2 | 4 | 6 | 8 | 10 |
|---|---|---|---|---|----|

❄ · · · · · · · 🔥

### BREAKFAST

_____:_____ AM/PM

FOODS:

HOW DO I FEEL?

### LUNCH

_____:_____ AM/PM

FOODS:

HOW DO I FEEL?

### DINNER

_____:_____ AM/PM

FOODS:

HOW DO I FEEL?

### SNACKS

_____:_____ AM/PM

FOODS:

HOW DO I FEEL?

## MOOD:

EXPLAIN WHY:

## NOTES:

..........................................................................
..........................................................................
..........................................................................
..........................................................................
..........................................................................

......../......../.............

## SLEEP:

............ HOURS OF SLEEP LAST NIGHT

## EXERCISE:

BIKE    SWIM    YOGA

WALK/HIKE    WEIGHTS    CARDIO

OTHER ACTIVITY:

............................................

TOTAL TIME
EXERCISING: ...........................

## WATER INTAKE:

8 oz   8 oz   8 oz   8 oz   8 oz

8 oz   8 oz   8 oz   8 oz   8 oz

## ENERGY:

0　2　4　6　8　10

## STRESS:

0　2　4　6　8　10

**BREAKFAST**　____:____AM/PM　FOODS:　HOW DO I FEEL?

**LUNCH**　____:____AM/PM　FOODS:　HOW DO I FEEL?

**DINNER**　____:____AM/PM　FOODS:　HOW DO I FEEL?

**SNACKS**　____:____AM/PM　FOODS:　HOW DO I FEEL?

## MOOD:

EXPLAIN WHY:

## NOTES:

......... / ........ / .............

## SLEEP:

🌙 ............. HOURS OF SLEEP LAST NIGHT

## EXERCISE:

BIKE   SWIM   YOGA

WALK/HIKE   WEIGHTS   CARDIO

OTHER ACTIVITY:

.....................................

TOTAL TIME
EXERCISING: .........................

## WATER INTAKE:

8 oz   8 oz   8 oz   8 oz   8 oz

8 oz   8 oz   8 oz   8 oz   8 oz

## ENERGY:

| 0 | 2 | 4 | 6 | 8 | 10 |
|---|---|---|---|---|----|

⊖ ......................... ⊕

## STRESS:

| 0 | 2 | 4 | 6 | 8 | 10 |
|---|---|---|---|---|----|

❋ ......................... 🔥

**BREAKFAST**
____:____ AM/PM
FOODS:

HOW DO I FEEL?

**LUNCH**
____:____ AM/PM
FOODS:

HOW DO I FEEL?

**DINNER**
____:____ AM/PM
FOODS:

HOW DO I FEEL?

**SNACKS**
____:____ AM/PM
FOODS:

HOW DO I FEEL?

## MOOD:

EXPLAIN WHY:

## NOTES:

...................................................
...................................................
...................................................
...................................................
...................................................

WHAT DO I EXPECT TO HAPPEN AFTER I FINISH THE 21 DAYS?

......................................................................................................
......................................................................................................
......................................................................................................
......................................................................................................

WHAT DO I WANT TO LEARN?

......................................................................................................
......................................................................................................
......................................................................................................
......................................................................................................

WHICH FOOD (IF ANY) DO I THINK WILL CAUSE ME PROBLEMS?
HOW DO I FEEL ABOUT THAT?

......................................................................................................
......................................................................................................
......................................................................................................
......................................................................................................

WHAT'S MY GAME PLAN IF I LEARN I NEED TO
ELIMINATE SOMETHING I EAT REGULARLY?

......................................................................................................
......................................................................................................
......................................................................................................
......................................................................................................

"Trust what your body is telling you."

-Erica

# CONGRATULATIONS,

## YOU WENT 21 DAYS SANS GLUTEN, DAIRY, AND MORE. IT'S A PRETTY BIG FEAT, NO? IT REALLY IS.

Which is why I am so happy to inform you that now it's time to add back in the foods you removed and track for potential triggers.

**Now, to do this successfully—you gotta follow these six steps:**

### STEP 1:

Choose one food item you eliminated to reintroduce into your diet on Day 22 and plan to reintroduce over a period of three days.

### STEP 2:

Be prepared to look for any changes to your skin, body, energy, sleep, and mood* over the three day period as those changes are signs the food you reintroduced is negatively affecting your body .

### STEP 3:

Make a plan to reintroduce the chosen food, being sure to reintroduce multiple variations of the food you plan to consume (e.g. for gluten - first day introduce bread for lunch, second day have pasta for dinner, third day eat grains for breakfast).

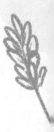

# YOU DID IT!

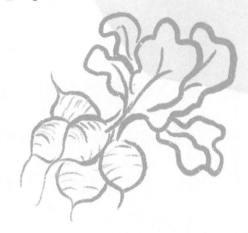

### STEP 4:

If the reintroduced food does not trigger you on the first day of reintroduction, continue eating variations of this food for the remaining two days and monitor for changes**. If it is obvious that the food you reintroduced triggers you the first day of reintroduction, stop eating immediately and do not eat that food or add in any new food item for the next two days, i.e. until the three day period is over.

### STEP 5:

On Day 25, reintroduce another food item you eliminated back into your diet over a period of three days to see if/how it affects your body.

### STEP 6:

Repeat Step 2–4 for all foods eliminated, reintroducing one food item at a time over a period of three days. Depending on the protocol you chose, the Trigger Tracker Process will take:

**Basic Elimination Diet:**
33 days (with reintroductions on Day 22, 25, 28, 31, ...)

**Liver-based Elimination Diet:**
39 days (with reintroduction on Day 22, 25, 28, 31, ...)

**Autoimmune Elimination Diet:**
54 days (with reintroductions on Day 22, 25, 28, 31, ...)

**Your Choice:**
21 days + (3 x # of items you will add back in) days

*Changes could include rashes, breakouts, slowed bowel movements, dips in energy, trouble falling or staying asleep, increased irritability, sinus pressure or runny nose, among many other things.

**Sometimes it takes up to 3 days to determine if a food triggers you / for changes in mood, energy, and skin to become obvious.

........./......../............

SLEEP:

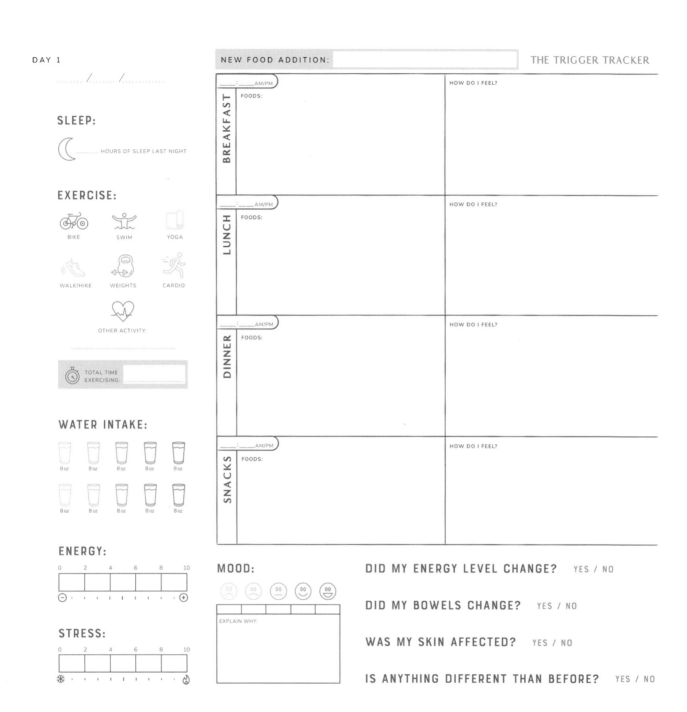

............. HOURS OF SLEEP LAST NIGHT

EXERCISE:

BIKE   SWIM   YOGA

WALK/HIKE   WEIGHTS   CARDIO

OTHER ACTIVITY:

.................................................

TOTAL TIME
EXERCISING:

WATER INTAKE:

8 oz   8 oz   8 oz   8 oz   8 oz

8 oz   8 oz   8 oz   8 oz   8 oz

ENERGY:

0   2   4   6   8   10

⊖ · ı ı ı ı ı ı · ⊕

STRESS:

0   2   4   6   8   10

❄ · ı ı ı ı ı ı · 🔥

NEW FOOD ADDITION:                                THE TRIGGER TRACKER

**BREAKFAST**   _____:_____ AM/PM
FOODS:                                    HOW DO I FEEL?

**LUNCH**   _____:_____ AM/PM
FOODS:                                    HOW DO I FEEL?

**DINNER**   _____:_____ AM/PM
FOODS:                                    HOW DO I FEEL?

**SNACKS**   _____:_____ AM/PM
FOODS:                                    HOW DO I FEEL?

MOOD:

EXPLAIN WHY:

DID MY ENERGY LEVEL CHANGE?   YES / NO

DID MY BOWELS CHANGE?   YES / NO

WAS MY SKIN AFFECTED?   YES / NO

IS ANYTHING DIFFERENT THAN BEFORE?   YES / NO

......... / ......... / ...............

## SLEEP:

🌙 ............. HOURS OF SLEEP LAST NIGHT

## EXERCISE:

BIKE     SWIM     YOGA

WALK/HIKE     WEIGHTS     CARDIO

OTHER ACTIVITY:

.......................................

⏱ TOTAL TIME
EXERCISING:

## WATER INTAKE:

8 oz    8 oz    8 oz    8 oz    8 oz

8 oz    8 oz    8 oz    8 oz    8 oz

## ENERGY:

| 0 | 2 | 4 | 6 | 8 | 10 |
|---|---|---|---|---|----|

⊖ · ' ' ' ' ' ' · ⊕

## STRESS:

| 0 | 2 | 4 | 6 | 8 | 10 |
|---|---|---|---|---|----|

❄ · ' ' ' ' ' ' · 🔥

---

NEW FOOD ADDITION: [                    ]          THE TRIGGER TRACKER

**BREAKFAST**

____:____ AM/PM
FOODS:

HOW DO I FEEL?

**LUNCH**

____:____ AM/PM
FOODS:

HOW DO I FEEL?

**DINNER**

____:____ AM/PM
FOODS:

HOW DO I FEEL?

**SNACKS**

____:____ AM/PM
FOODS:

HOW DO I FEEL?

## MOOD:

EXPLAIN WHY:

DID MY ENERGY LEVEL CHANGE?    YES / NO

DID MY BOWELS CHANGE?    YES / NO

WAS MY SKIN AFFECTED?    YES / NO

IS ANYTHING DIFFERENT THAN BEFORE?    YES / NO

......... / ........ / ...............

## SLEEP:

.............. HOURS OF SLEEP LAST NIGHT

## EXERCISE:

BIKE    SWIM    YOGA

WALK/HIKE    WEIGHTS    CARDIO

OTHER ACTIVITY:
.................................

TOTAL TIME
EXERCISING: ..........................

## WATER INTAKE:

8 oz    8 oz    8 oz    8 oz    8 oz

8 oz    8 oz    8 oz    8 oz    8 oz

## ENERGY:

0    2    4    6    8    10

⊖ · · · · · · · · · ⊕

## STRESS:

0    2    4    6    8    10

❄ · · · · · · · · · 🔥

NEW FOOD ADDITION: _____    THE TRIGGER TRACKER

**BREAKFAST**  ____:____ AM/PM    FOODS:    HOW DO I FEEL?

**LUNCH**  ____:____ AM/PM    FOODS:    HOW DO I FEEL?

**DINNER**  ____:____ AM/PM    FOODS:    HOW DO I FEEL?

**SNACKS**  ____:____ AM/PM    FOODS:    HOW DO I FEEL?

## MOOD:

😟  🙁  😐  🙂  😄

EXPLAIN WHY:

DID MY ENERGY LEVEL CHANGE?    YES / NO

DID MY BOWELS CHANGE?    YES / NO

WAS MY SKIN AFFECTED?    YES / NO

IS ANYTHING DIFFERENT THAN BEFORE?    YES / NO

HOW DID I FEEL EATING THIS FOOD ITEM?

..................................................................................................................................
..................................................................................................................................
..................................................................................................................................
..................................................................................................................................

WHAT DID I LEARN ABOUT MYSELF AND MY BODY DURING THIS PROCESS?

..................................................................................................................................
..................................................................................................................................
..................................................................................................................................

WHAT DO I FIND MOST INTERESTING ABOUT THIS PROCESS?

..................................................................................................................................
..................................................................................................................................
..................................................................................................................................
..................................................................................................................................

WHAT IS MY BIGGEST TAKEAWAY FROM THIS JOURNEY?

..................................................................................................................................
..................................................................................................................................
..................................................................................................................................
..................................................................................................................................
..................................................................................................................................

WILL I CONTINUE TO EAT THIS FOOD?  YES  /  NO

NEW FOOD ADDITION:

......... / ......... / .............

**SLEEP:**

........... HOURS OF SLEEP LAST NIGHT

**EXERCISE:**

BIKE          SWIM          YOGA

WALK/HIKE     WEIGHTS       CARDIO

OTHER ACTIVITY:

...................................................

TOTAL TIME
EXERCISING:

**WATER INTAKE:**

8 oz   8 oz   8 oz   8 oz   8 oz

8 oz   8 oz   8 oz   8 oz   8 oz

**ENERGY:**

0    2    4    6    8    10
⊖ · ' ' ' ' ' ' · ⊕

**STRESS:**

0    2    4    6    8    10
☀ · ' ' ' ' ' ' · 🔥

**BREAKFAST**

_____:_____AM/PM
FOODS:

HOW DO I FEEL?

**LUNCH**

_____:_____AM/PM
FOODS:

HOW DO I FEEL?

**DINNER**

_____:_____AM/PM
FOODS:

HOW DO I FEEL?

**SNACKS**

_____:_____AM/PM
FOODS:

HOW DO I FEEL?

**MOOD:**

EXPLAIN WHY:

**DID MY ENERGY LEVEL CHANGE?**   YES / NO

**DID MY BOWELS CHANGE?**   YES / NO

**WAS MY SKIN AFFECTED?**   YES / NO

**IS ANYTHING DIFFERENT THAN BEFORE?**   YES / NO

......... / ......... / .........

NEW FOOD ADDITION: [                    ]          THE TRIGGER TRACKER

## SLEEP:

☾ ............. HOURS OF SLEEP LAST NIGHT

## EXERCISE:

BIKE        SWIM        YOGA

WALK/HIKE   WEIGHTS     CARDIO

OTHER ACTIVITY:
.................................................

TOTAL TIME
EXERCISING: .................................

## WATER INTAKE:

8 oz   8 oz   8 oz   8 oz   8 oz

8 oz   8 oz   8 oz   8 oz   8 oz

## ENERGY:

0    2    4    6    8    10

⊖ · · · · · · · · · · ⊕

## STRESS:

0    2    4    6    8    10

❊ · · · · · · · · · · 🔥

**BREAKFAST**
_____:_____ AM/PM
FOODS:

HOW DO I FEEL?

**LUNCH**
_____:_____ AM/PM
FOODS:

HOW DO I FEEL?

**DINNER**
_____:_____ AM/PM
FOODS:

HOW DO I FEEL?

**SNACKS**
_____:_____ AM/PM
FOODS:

HOW DO I FEEL?

## MOOD:

☹ 🙁 😐 🙂 😄

EXPLAIN WHY:

DID MY ENERGY LEVEL CHANGE?   YES / NO

DID MY BOWELS CHANGE?   YES / NO

WAS MY SKIN AFFECTED?   YES / NO

IS ANYTHING DIFFERENT THAN BEFORE?   YES / NO

........ / ........ / ..............

## SLEEP:

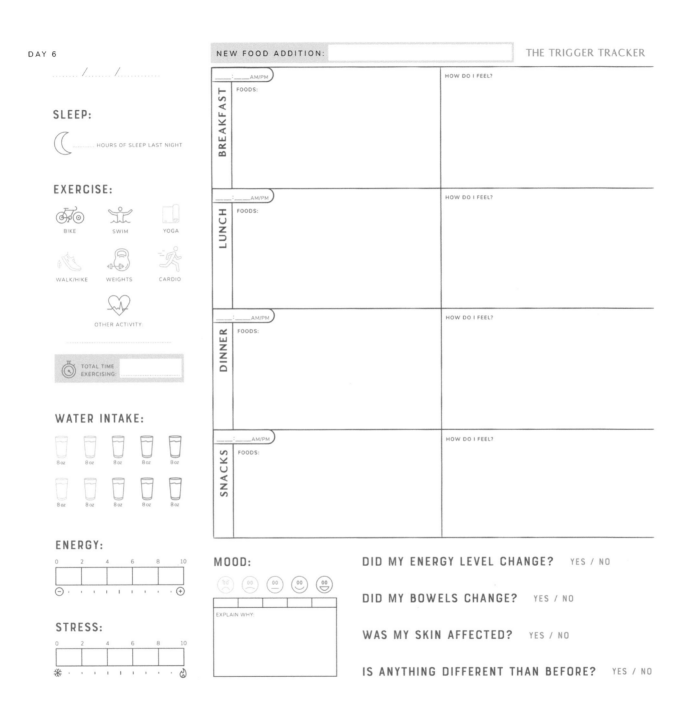

............ HOURS OF SLEEP LAST NIGHT

## EXERCISE:

BIKE          SWIM          YOGA

WALK/HIKE     WEIGHTS       CARDIO

OTHER ACTIVITY:

..............................................

TOTAL TIME
EXERCISING:

## WATER INTAKE:

8 oz   8 oz   8 oz   8 oz   8 oz

8 oz   8 oz   8 oz   8 oz   8 oz

## ENERGY:

0   2   4   6   8   10

⊖ · · · · · · · · · ⊕

## STRESS:

0   2   4   6   8   10

❄ · · · · · · · · · 🔥

**BREAKFAST**   _____:_____ AM/PM     HOW DO I FEEL?
FOODS:

**LUNCH**   _____:_____ AM/PM     HOW DO I FEEL?
FOODS:

**DINNER**   _____:_____ AM/PM     HOW DO I FEEL?
FOODS:

**SNACKS**   _____:_____ AM/PM     HOW DO I FEEL?
FOODS:

## MOOD:

EXPLAIN WHY:

**DID MY ENERGY LEVEL CHANGE?**   YES / NO

**DID MY BOWELS CHANGE?**   YES / NO

**WAS MY SKIN AFFECTED?**   YES / NO

**IS ANYTHING DIFFERENT THAN BEFORE?**   YES / NO

HOW DID I FEEL EATING THIS FOOD ITEM?

......................................................................................................................................

......................................................................................................................................

......................................................................................................................................

......................................................................................................................................

WHAT DID I LEARN ABOUT MYSELF AND MY BODY DURING THIS PROCESS?

......................................................................................................................................

......................................................................................................................................

......................................................................................................................................

WHAT DO I FIND MOST INTERESTING ABOUT THIS PROCESS?

......................................................................................................................................

......................................................................................................................................

......................................................................................................................................

......................................................................................................................................

WHAT IS MY BIGGEST TAKEAWAY FROM THIS JOURNEY?

......................................................................................................................................

......................................................................................................................................

......................................................................................................................................

......................................................................................................................................

......................................................................................................................................

WILL I CONTINUE TO EAT THIS FOOD?  YES  /  NO

........ / ........ / ...........

## SLEEP:

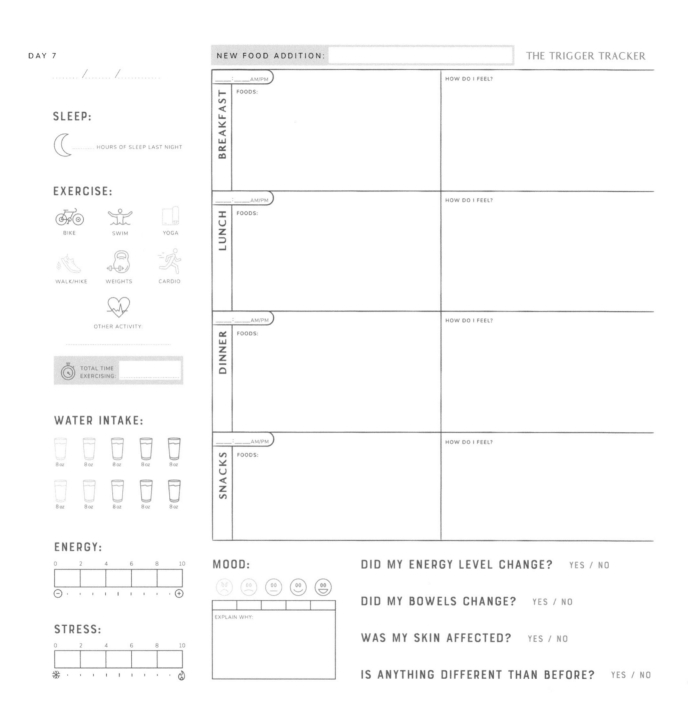

............... HOURS OF SLEEP LAST NIGHT

## EXERCISE:

BIKE    SWIM    YOGA

WALK/HIKE    WEIGHTS    CARDIO

OTHER ACTIVITY:

...........................................

TOTAL TIME
EXERCISING: ...........................

## WATER INTAKE:

8 oz  8 oz  8 oz  8 oz  8 oz

8 oz  8 oz  8 oz  8 oz  8 oz

## ENERGY:

0    2    4    6    8    10

⊖ · · · · · · · · · ⊕

## STRESS:

0    2    4    6    8    10

❄ · · · · · · · · · 🔥

NEW FOOD ADDITION:                                    THE TRIGGER TRACKER

**BREAKFAST**
_____:_____AM/PM
FOODS:                                                HOW DO I FEEL?

**LUNCH**
_____:_____AM/PM
FOODS:                                                HOW DO I FEEL?

**DINNER**
_____:_____AM/PM
FOODS:                                                HOW DO I FEEL?

**SNACKS**
_____:_____AM/PM
FOODS:                                                HOW DO I FEEL?

## MOOD:

EXPLAIN WHY:

**DID MY ENERGY LEVEL CHANGE?**   YES / NO

**DID MY BOWELS CHANGE?**   YES / NO

**WAS MY SKIN AFFECTED?**   YES / NO

**IS ANYTHING DIFFERENT THAN BEFORE?**   YES / NO

.......... / .......... / ..........

## SLEEP:

( .......... HOURS OF SLEEP LAST NIGHT

## EXERCISE:

BIKE          SWIM          YOGA

WALK/HIKE     WEIGHTS       CARDIO

OTHER ACTIVITY:

..........................................................

TOTAL TIME EXERCISING: _____

## WATER INTAKE:

8 oz   8 oz   8 oz   8 oz   8 oz

8 oz   8 oz   8 oz   8 oz   8 oz

## ENERGY:

0   2   4   6   8   10

⊖ · · · · · · · · · ⊕

## STRESS:

0   2   4   6   8   10

❄ · · · · · · · · · ⏱

**NEW FOOD ADDITION:** _____          THE TRIGGER TRACKER

### BREAKFAST
____:____ AM/PM
FOODS:

HOW DO I FEEL?

### LUNCH
____:____ AM/PM
FOODS:

HOW DO I FEEL?

### DINNER
____:____ AM/PM
FOODS:

HOW DO I FEEL?

### SNACKS
____:____ AM/PM
FOODS:

HOW DO I FEEL?

## MOOD:

😟 😕 😐 🙂 😄

EXPLAIN WHY:

**DID MY ENERGY LEVEL CHANGE?**   YES / NO

**DID MY BOWELS CHANGE?**   YES / NO

**WAS MY SKIN AFFECTED?**   YES / NO

**IS ANYTHING DIFFERENT THAN BEFORE?**   YES / NO

........ / ........ / ........

## SLEEP:

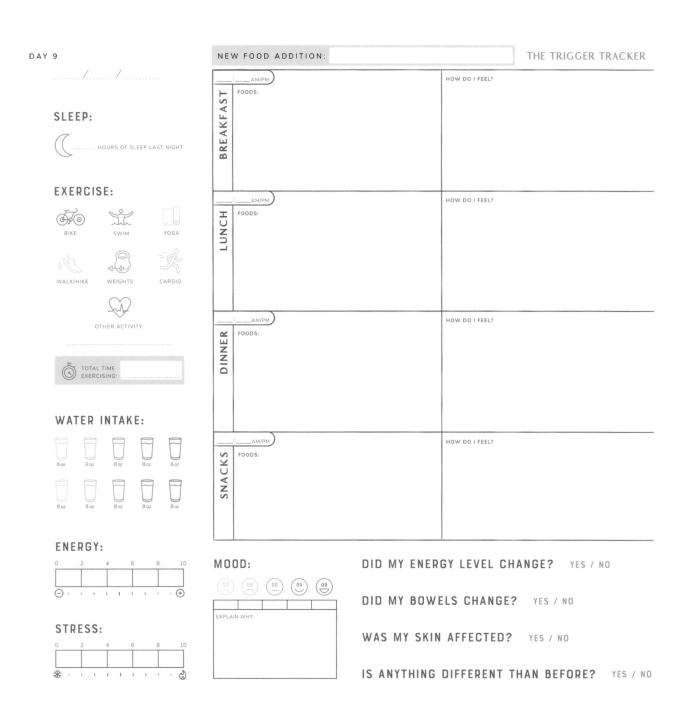

........ HOURS OF SLEEP LAST NIGHT

## EXERCISE:

BIKE     SWIM     YOGA

WALK/HIKE     WEIGHTS     CARDIO

OTHER ACTIVITY:

........................................

TOTAL TIME
EXERCISING: ........................

## WATER INTAKE:

8 oz   8 oz   8 oz   8 oz   8 oz

8 oz   8 oz   8 oz   8 oz   8 oz

## ENERGY:

0     2     4     6     8     10

⊖ · ' ' ' ' ' ' ' ⊕

## STRESS:

0     2     4     6     8     10

❋ · ' ' ' ' ' ' ' 🔥

NEW FOOD ADDITION: [                    ]     THE TRIGGER TRACKER

**BREAKFAST**   ____:____ AM/PM     HOW DO I FEEL?
FOODS:

**LUNCH**   ____:____ AM/PM     HOW DO I FEEL?
FOODS:

**DINNER**   ____:____ AM/PM     HOW DO I FEEL?
FOODS:

**SNACKS**   ____:____ AM/PM     HOW DO I FEEL?
FOODS:

## MOOD:

EXPLAIN WHY:

DID MY ENERGY LEVEL CHANGE?   YES / NO

DID MY BOWELS CHANGE?   YES / NO

WAS MY SKIN AFFECTED?   YES / NO

IS ANYTHING DIFFERENT THAN BEFORE?   YES / NO

HOW DID I FEEL EATING THIS FOOD ITEM?

..................................................................................................................................
..................................................................................................................................
..................................................................................................................................
..................................................................................................................................

WHAT DID I LEARN ABOUT MYSELF AND MY BODY DURING THIS PROCESS?

..................................................................................................................................
..................................................................................................................................
..................................................................................................................................

WHAT DO I FIND MOST INTERESTING ABOUT THIS PROCESS?

..................................................................................................................................
..................................................................................................................................
..................................................................................................................................
..................................................................................................................................

WHAT IS MY BIGGEST TAKEAWAY FROM THIS JOURNEY?

..................................................................................................................................
..................................................................................................................................
..................................................................................................................................
..................................................................................................................................
..................................................................................................................................
..................................................................................................................................

WILL I CONTINUE TO EAT THIS FOOD?  YES  /  NO

......../......../...............

## SLEEP:

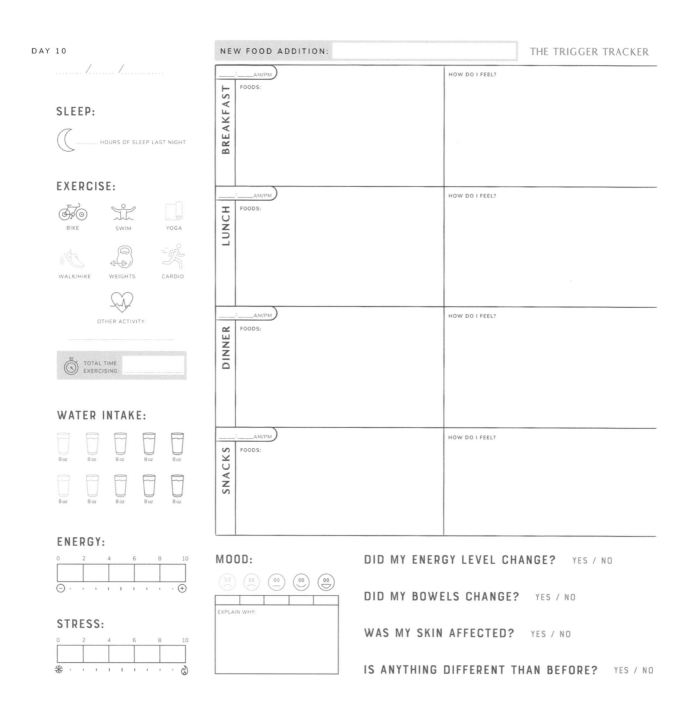

........... HOURS OF SLEEP LAST NIGHT

## EXERCISE:

BIKE    SWIM    YOGA

WALK/HIKE    WEIGHTS    CARDIO

OTHER ACTIVITY:

......................................................

TOTAL TIME
EXERCISING: ....................................

## WATER INTAKE:

8 oz    8 oz    8 oz    8 oz    8 oz

8 oz    8 oz    8 oz    8 oz    8 oz

## ENERGY:

0    2    4    6    8    10

⊖ · · · · · · · · · ⊕

## STRESS:

0    2    4    6    8    10

✳ · · · · · · · · · 🔥

**BREAKFAST**

_____:_____ AM/PM

FOODS:

HOW DO I FEEL?

**LUNCH**

_____:_____ AM/PM

FOODS:

HOW DO I FEEL?

**DINNER**

_____:_____ AM/PM

FOODS:

HOW DO I FEEL?

**SNACKS**

_____:_____ AM/PM

FOODS:

HOW DO I FEEL?

## MOOD:

EXPLAIN WHY:

**DID MY ENERGY LEVEL CHANGE?**    YES / NO

**DID MY BOWELS CHANGE?**    YES / NO

**WAS MY SKIN AFFECTED?**    YES / NO

**IS ANYTHING DIFFERENT THAN BEFORE?**    YES / NO

.........../........./...........

**SLEEP:**

........... HOURS OF SLEEP LAST NIGHT

**EXERCISE:**

BIKE          SWIM          YOGA

WALK/HIKE     WEIGHTS       CARDIO

OTHER ACTIVITY:

...................................................

TOTAL TIME
EXERCISING:

**WATER INTAKE:**

8 oz   8 oz   8 oz   8 oz   8 oz

8 oz   8 oz   8 oz   8 oz   8 oz

**ENERGY:**

| 0 | 2 | 4 | 6 | 8 | 10 |

$\ominus$ · · · · · · · · · $\oplus$

**STRESS:**

| 0 | 2 | 4 | 6 | 8 | 10 |

❄ · · · · · · · · · 🔥

**BREAKFAST**

_____:_____ AM/PM

FOODS:

HOW DO I FEEL?

**LUNCH**

_____:_____ AM/PM

FOODS:

HOW DO I FEEL?

**DINNER**

_____:_____ AM/PM

FOODS:

HOW DO I FEEL?

**SNACKS**

_____:_____ AM/PM

FOODS:

HOW DO I FEEL?

**MOOD:**

EXPLAIN WHY:

**DID MY ENERGY LEVEL CHANGE?** YES / NO

**DID MY BOWELS CHANGE?** YES / NO

**WAS MY SKIN AFFECTED?** YES / NO

**IS ANYTHING DIFFERENT THAN BEFORE?** YES / NO

......... / ......... / .............

## SLEEP:

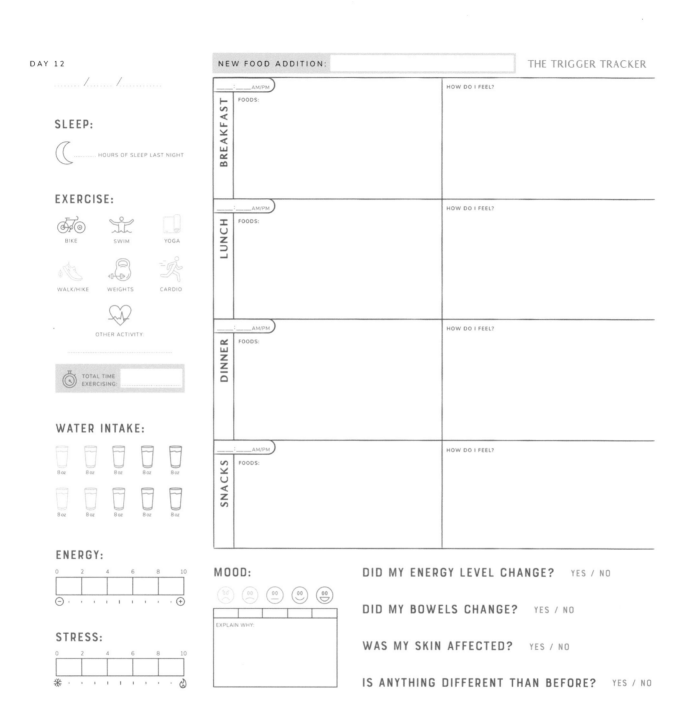

........... HOURS OF SLEEP LAST NIGHT

## EXERCISE:

BIKE          SWIM          YOGA

WALK/HIKE     WEIGHTS       CARDIO

OTHER ACTIVITY:

........................................................

TOTAL TIME
EXERCISING: ...........................

## WATER INTAKE:

8 oz    8 oz    8 oz    8 oz    8 oz

8 oz    8 oz    8 oz    8 oz    8 oz

## ENERGY:

0    2    4    6    8    10

⊖ · · · · · · · · · ⊕

## STRESS:

0    2    4    6    8    10

❋ · · · · · · · · · 🔥

---

NEW FOOD ADDITION:

THE TRIGGER TRACKER

**BREAKFAST**
_____:_____ AM/PM
FOODS:

HOW DO I FEEL?

**LUNCH**
_____:_____ AM/PM
FOODS:

HOW DO I FEEL?

**DINNER**
_____:_____ AM/PM
FOODS:

HOW DO I FEEL?

**SNACKS**
_____:_____ AM/PM
FOODS:

HOW DO I FEEL?

## MOOD:

EXPLAIN WHY:

DID MY ENERGY LEVEL CHANGE?   YES / NO

DID MY BOWELS CHANGE?   YES / NO

WAS MY SKIN AFFECTED?   YES / NO

IS ANYTHING DIFFERENT THAN BEFORE?   YES / NO

HOW DID I FEEL EATING THIS FOOD ITEM?

.................................................................................................................................................

.................................................................................................................................................

.................................................................................................................................................

.................................................................................................................................................

WHAT DID I LEARN ABOUT MYSELF AND MY BODY DURING THIS PROCESS?

.................................................................................................................................................

.................................................................................................................................................

.................................................................................................................................................

WHAT DO I FIND MOST INTERESTING ABOUT THIS PROCESS?

.................................................................................................................................................

.................................................................................................................................................

.................................................................................................................................................

WHAT IS MY BIGGEST TAKEAWAY FROM THIS JOURNEY?

.................................................................................................................................................

.................................................................................................................................................

.................................................................................................................................................

.................................................................................................................................................

.................................................................................................................................................

WILL I CONTINUE TO EAT THIS FOOD?  YES / NO

........ / ........ / ................

## SLEEP:

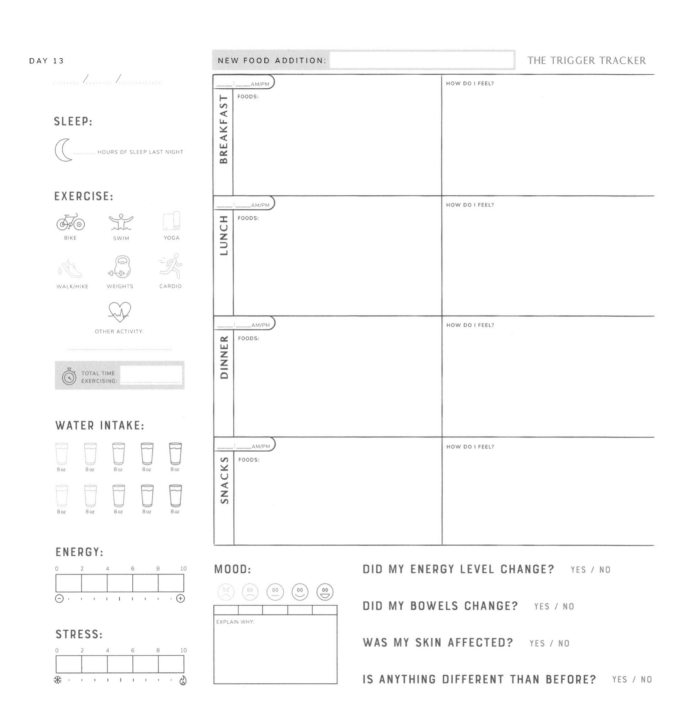

............... HOURS OF SLEEP LAST NIGHT

## EXERCISE:

BIKE SWIM YOGA

WALK/HIKE WEIGHTS CARDIO

OTHER ACTIVITY:

...............................................

TOTAL TIME
EXERCISING:

## WATER INTAKE:

8 oz    8 oz    8 oz    8 oz    8 oz

8 oz    8 oz    8 oz    8 oz    8 oz

## ENERGY:

0    2    4    6    8    10

⊖ · · · · · · · · · · ⊕

## STRESS:

0    2    4    6    8    10

❄ · · · · · · · · · · 🔥

NEW FOOD ADDITION: _____

THE TRIGGER TRACKER

**BREAKFAST**
____:____ AM/PM
FOODS:
HOW DO I FEEL?

**LUNCH**
____:____ AM/PM
FOODS:
HOW DO I FEEL?

**DINNER**
____:____ AM/PM
FOODS:
HOW DO I FEEL?

**SNACKS**
____:____ AM/PM
FOODS:
HOW DO I FEEL?

## MOOD:

EXPLAIN WHY:

DID MY ENERGY LEVEL CHANGE?   YES / NO

DID MY BOWELS CHANGE?   YES / NO

WAS MY SKIN AFFECTED?   YES / NO

IS ANYTHING DIFFERENT THAN BEFORE?   YES / NO

.............. / ............ / ..............

**NEW FOOD ADDITION:** |_____| THE TRIGGER TRACKER

## SLEEP:

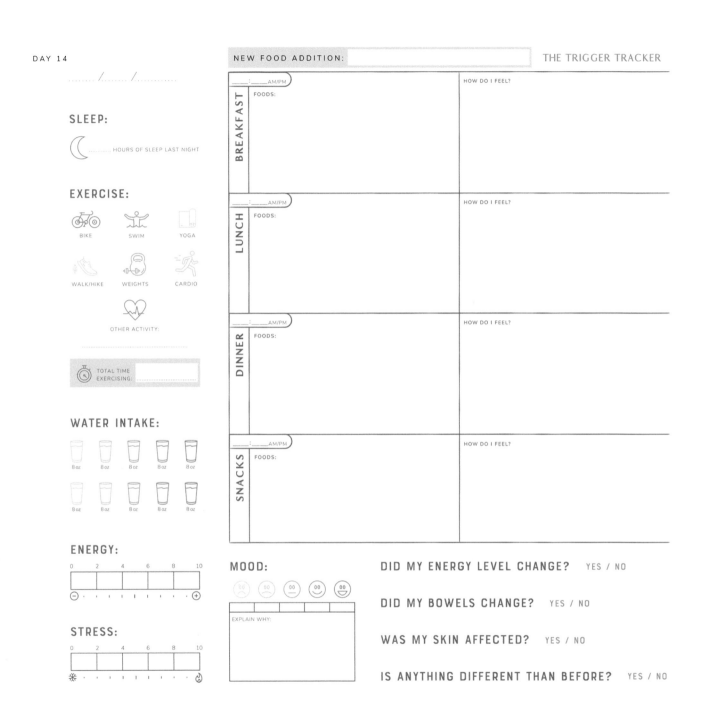

.............. HOURS OF SLEEP LAST NIGHT

## EXERCISE:

BIKE | SWIM | YOGA

WALK/HIKE | WEIGHTS | CARDIO

OTHER ACTIVITY:

..................................................

TOTAL TIME EXERCISING: ..................................

## WATER INTAKE:

8 oz | 8 oz | 8 oz | 8 oz | 8 oz

8 oz | 8 oz | 8 oz | 8 oz | 8 oz

## ENERGY:

0  2  4  6  8  10

⊖ · · · · · · · · · · ⊕

## STRESS:

0  2  4  6  8  10

❄ · · · · · · · · · · 🔥

**BREAKFAST**  _____:_____ AM/PM  FOODS:  HOW DO I FEEL?

**LUNCH**  _____:_____ AM/PM  FOODS:  HOW DO I FEEL?

**DINNER**  _____:_____ AM/PM  FOODS:  HOW DO I FEEL?

**SNACKS**  _____:_____ AM/PM  FOODS:  HOW DO I FEEL?

## MOOD:

EXPLAIN WHY:

DID MY ENERGY LEVEL CHANGE?  YES / NO

DID MY BOWELS CHANGE?  YES / NO

WAS MY SKIN AFFECTED?  YES / NO

IS ANYTHING DIFFERENT THAN BEFORE?  YES / NO

........./.........../.............

## SLEEP:

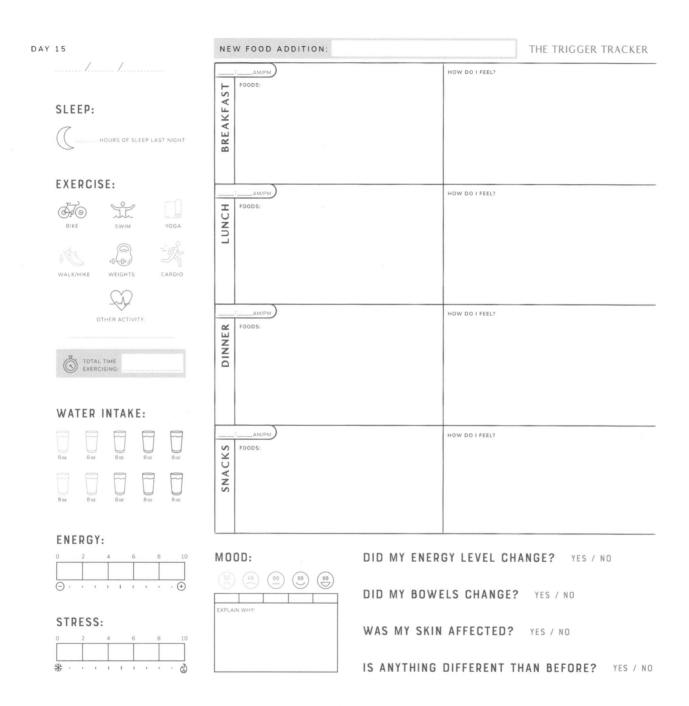

............... HOURS OF SLEEP LAST NIGHT

## EXERCISE:

BIKE  SWIM  YOGA

WALK/HIKE  WEIGHTS  CARDIO

OTHER ACTIVITY:

..............................................

TOTAL TIME
EXERCISING:

## WATER INTAKE:

8 oz  8 oz  8 oz  8 oz  8 oz

8 oz  8 oz  8 oz  8 oz  8 oz

## ENERGY:

0   2   4   6   8   10

⊖ · · · · · · · · · ⊕

## STRESS:

0   2   4   6   8   10

❄ · · · · · · · · · 🔥

**NEW FOOD ADDITION:**

THE TRIGGER TRACKER

**BREAKFAST**  ____:____ AM/PM   HOW DO I FEEL?
FOODS:

**LUNCH**  ____:____ AM/PM   HOW DO I FEEL?
FOODS:

**DINNER**  ____:____ AM/PM   HOW DO I FEEL?
FOODS:

**SNACKS**  ____:____ AM/PM   HOW DO I FEEL?
FOODS:

## MOOD:

EXPLAIN WHY:

**DID MY ENERGY LEVEL CHANGE?**   YES / NO

**DID MY BOWELS CHANGE?**   YES / NO

**WAS MY SKIN AFFECTED?**   YES / NO

**IS ANYTHING DIFFERENT THAN BEFORE?**   YES / NO

HOW DID I FEEL EATING THIS FOOD ITEM?

...........................................................................................................

...........................................................................................................

...........................................................................................................

...........................................................................................................

WHAT DID I LEARN ABOUT MYSELF AND MY BODY DURING THIS PROCESS?

...........................................................................................................

...........................................................................................................

...........................................................................................................

WHAT DO I FIND MOST INTERESTING ABOUT THIS PROCESS?

...........................................................................................................

...........................................................................................................

...........................................................................................................

WHAT IS MY BIGGEST TAKEAWAY FROM THIS JOURNEY?

...........................................................................................................

...........................................................................................................

...........................................................................................................

...........................................................................................................

...........................................................................................................

...........................................................................................................

WILL I CONTINUE TO EAT THIS FOOD?  YES  /  NO

........ / ........ / ............

**SLEEP:**

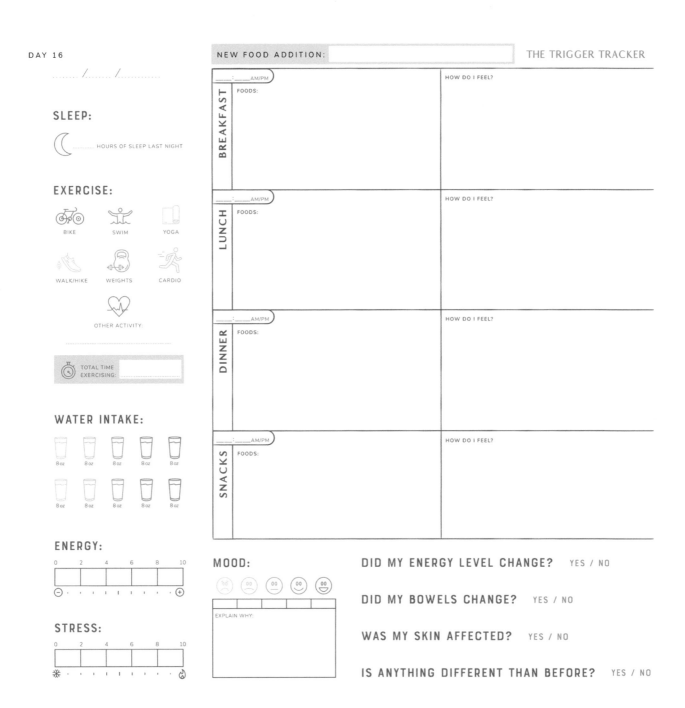

........ HOURS OF SLEEP LAST NIGHT

**EXERCISE:**

BIKE  SWIM  YOGA

WALK/HIKE  WEIGHTS  CARDIO

OTHER ACTIVITY:

........................................

TOTAL TIME
EXERCISING:

**WATER INTAKE:**

8 oz  8 oz  8 oz  8 oz  8 oz

8 oz  8 oz  8 oz  8 oz  8 oz

**ENERGY:**

0   2   4   6   8   10

$\ominus$ . . . . . . . . . . $\oplus$

**STRESS:**

0   2   4   6   8   10

❋ . . . . . . . . . . 🔥

NEW FOOD ADDITION:

THE TRIGGER TRACKER

**BREAKFAST**

_____:_____ AM/PM

FOODS:

HOW DO I FEEL?

**LUNCH**

_____:_____ AM/PM

FOODS:

HOW DO I FEEL?

**DINNER**

_____:_____ AM/PM

FOODS:

HOW DO I FEEL?

**SNACKS**

_____:_____ AM/PM

FOODS:

HOW DO I FEEL?

**MOOD:**

EXPLAIN WHY:

DID MY ENERGY LEVEL CHANGE?   YES / NO

DID MY BOWELS CHANGE?   YES / NO

WAS MY SKIN AFFECTED?   YES / NO

IS ANYTHING DIFFERENT THAN BEFORE?   YES / NO

........../........./..........

## SLEEP:

🌙 .......... HOURS OF SLEEP LAST NIGHT

## EXERCISE:

BIKE   SWIM   YOGA

WALK/HIKE   WEIGHTS   CARDIO

OTHER ACTIVITY:
................................................

⏱ TOTAL TIME
EXERCISING: ....................................

## WATER INTAKE:

8 oz   8 oz   8 oz   8 oz   8 oz

8 oz   8 oz   8 oz   8 oz   8 oz

## ENERGY:

0   2   4   6   8   10

⊖ · · · · · · · · · ⊕

## STRESS:

0   2   4   6   8   10

✳ · · · · · · · · · 🔥

**BREAKFAST** _____:_____ AM/PM
FOODS:

HOW DO I FEEL?

**LUNCH** _____:_____ AM/PM
FOODS:

HOW DO I FEEL?

**DINNER** _____:_____ AM/PM
FOODS:

HOW DO I FEEL?

**SNACKS** _____:_____ AM/PM
FOODS:

HOW DO I FEEL?

## MOOD:

😣 🙁 😐 🙂 😀

EXPLAIN WHY:

DID MY ENERGY LEVEL CHANGE?   YES / NO

DID MY BOWELS CHANGE?   YES / NO

WAS MY SKIN AFFECTED?   YES / NO

IS ANYTHING DIFFERENT THAN BEFORE?   YES / NO

......... / ......... / ...............

## SLEEP:

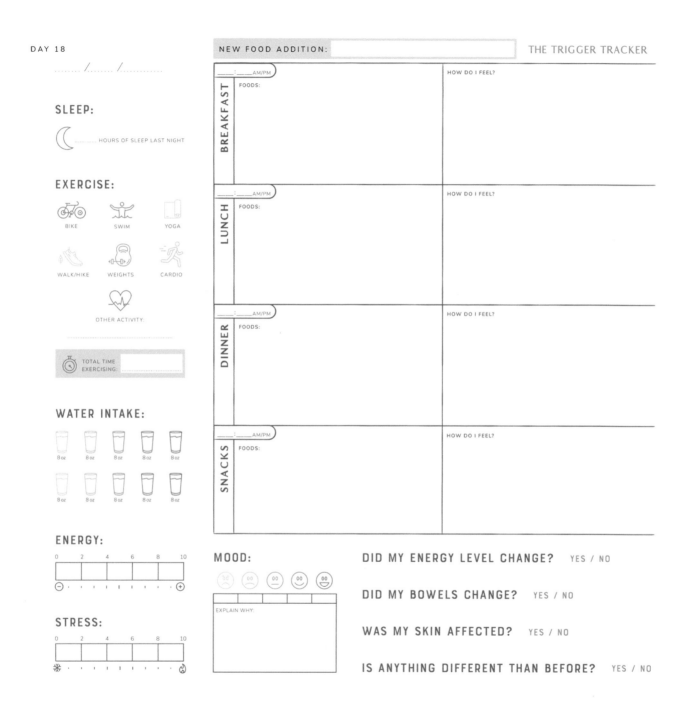

.......... HOURS OF SLEEP LAST NIGHT

## EXERCISE:

BIKE        SWIM        YOGA

WALK/HIKE   WEIGHTS     CARDIO

OTHER ACTIVITY:

.............................................

TOTAL TIME
EXERCISING:

## WATER INTAKE:

8 oz   8 oz   8 oz   8 oz   8 oz

8 oz   8 oz   8 oz   8 oz   8 oz

## ENERGY:

0   2   4   6   8   10

⊖ · · · · · · · · · ⊕

## STRESS:

0   2   4   6   8   10

❄ · · · · · · · · · 🔥

NEW FOOD ADDITION:                                        THE TRIGGER TRACKER

**BREAKFAST**
_____:_____ AM/PM
FOODS:                                  HOW DO I FEEL?

**LUNCH**
_____:_____ AM/PM
FOODS:                                  HOW DO I FEEL?

**DINNER**
_____:_____ AM/PM
FOODS:                                  HOW DO I FEEL?

**SNACKS**
_____:_____ AM/PM
FOODS:                                  HOW DO I FEEL?

MOOD:

EXPLAIN WHY:

DID MY ENERGY LEVEL CHANGE?    YES / NO

DID MY BOWELS CHANGE?    YES / NO

WAS MY SKIN AFFECTED?    YES / NO

IS ANYTHING DIFFERENT THAN BEFORE?    YES / NO

HOW DID I FEEL EATING THIS FOOD ITEM?

..................................................................................................................................

..................................................................................................................................

..................................................................................................................................

..................................................................................................................................

WHAT DID I LEARN ABOUT MYSELF AND MY BODY DURING THIS PROCESS?

..................................................................................................................................

..................................................................................................................................

..................................................................................................................................

WHAT DO I FIND MOST INTERESTING ABOUT THIS PROCESS?

..................................................................................................................................

..................................................................................................................................

..................................................................................................................................

WHAT IS MY BIGGEST TAKEAWAY FROM THIS JOURNEY?

..................................................................................................................................

..................................................................................................................................

..................................................................................................................................

..................................................................................................................................

..................................................................................................................................

WILL I CONTINUE TO EAT THIS FOOD?  YES / NO

......... / .......... / .............

## SLEEP:

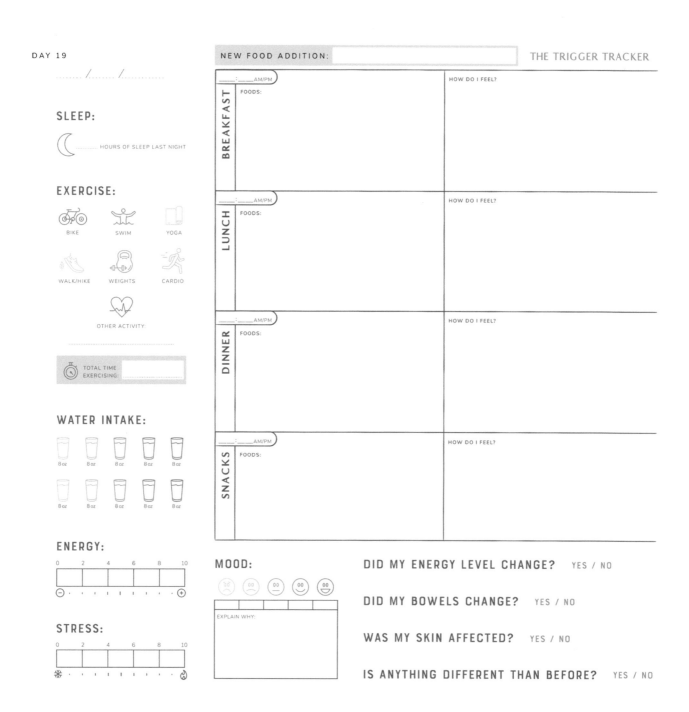

....... HOURS OF SLEEP LAST NIGHT

## EXERCISE:

BIKE  SWIM  YOGA

WALK/HIKE  WEIGHTS  CARDIO

OTHER ACTIVITY:

.................................................

TOTAL TIME
EXERCISING:

## WATER INTAKE:

8 oz  8 oz  8 oz  8 oz  8 oz

8 oz  8 oz  8 oz  8 oz  8 oz

## ENERGY:

0    2    4    6    8    10

⊖ · · · · · · · · · ⊕

## STRESS:

0    2    4    6    8    10

❄ · · · · · · · · · 🔥

NEW FOOD ADDITION:

THE TRIGGER TRACKER

**BREAKFAST**
____:____ AM/PM
FOODS:

HOW DO I FEEL?

**LUNCH**
____:____ AM/PM
FOODS:

HOW DO I FEEL?

**DINNER**
____:____ AM/PM
FOODS:

HOW DO I FEEL?

**SNACKS**
____:____ AM/PM
FOODS:

HOW DO I FEEL?

## MOOD:

EXPLAIN WHY:

DID MY ENERGY LEVEL CHANGE?  YES / NO

DID MY BOWELS CHANGE?  YES / NO

WAS MY SKIN AFFECTED?  YES / NO

IS ANYTHING DIFFERENT THAN BEFORE?  YES / NO

........../........./.............

**SLEEP:**

☾ ............... HOURS OF SLEEP LAST NIGHT

**EXERCISE:**

BIKE          SWIM          YOGA

WALK/HIKE    WEIGHTS      CARDIO

OTHER ACTIVITY:

.................................................

TOTAL TIME
EXERCISING: ...........................................

**WATER INTAKE:**

8oz   8oz   8oz   8oz   8oz

8oz   8oz   8oz   8oz   8oz

**ENERGY:**

0    2    4    6    8    10

⊖ · · · · · · · · · ⊕

**STRESS:**

0    2    4    6    8    10

✳ · · · · · · · · · 🌀

**NEW FOOD ADDITION:** _____          THE TRIGGER TRACKER

**BREAKFAST**

_____:_____AM/PM
FOODS:

HOW DO I FEEL?

**LUNCH**

_____:_____AM/PM
FOODS:

HOW DO I FEEL?

**DINNER**

_____:_____AM/PM
FOODS:

HOW DO I FEEL?

**SNACKS**

_____:_____AM/PM
FOODS:

HOW DO I FEEL?

**MOOD:**

EXPLAIN WHY:

**DID MY ENERGY LEVEL CHANGE?**   YES / NO

**DID MY BOWELS CHANGE?**   YES / NO

**WAS MY SKIN AFFECTED?**   YES / NO

**IS ANYTHING DIFFERENT THAN BEFORE?**   YES / NO

........./........./...............

**SLEEP:**

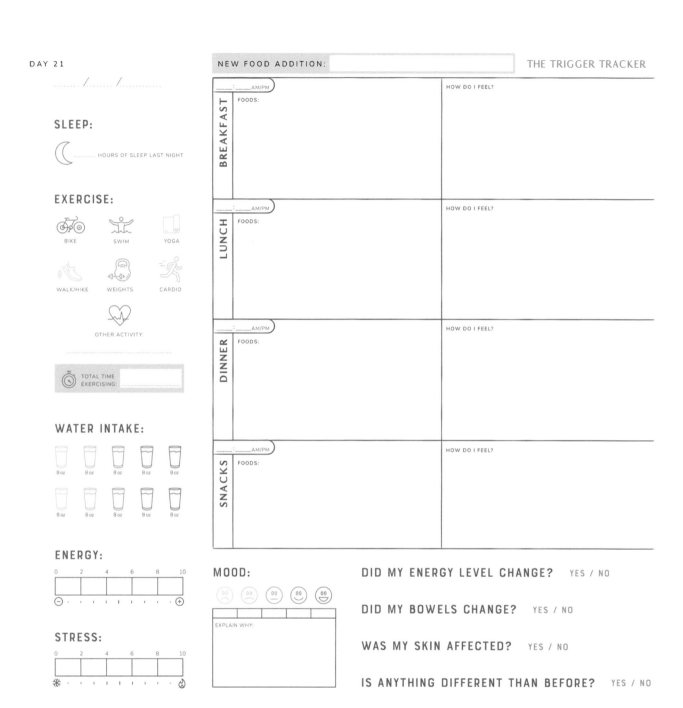

............... HOURS OF SLEEP LAST NIGHT

**EXERCISE:**

BIKE    SWIM    YOGA

WALK/HIKE    WEIGHTS    CARDIO

OTHER ACTIVITY

...........................................

TOTAL TIME
EXERCISING:

**WATER INTAKE:**

8 oz    8 oz    8 oz    8 oz    8 oz

8 oz    8 oz    8 oz    8 oz    8 oz

**ENERGY:**

0    2    4    6    8    10

⊖ · · · · · · · · ⊕

**STRESS:**

0    2    4    6    8    10

❄ · · · · · · · · 🔥

NEW FOOD ADDITION:

THE TRIGGER TRACKER

_____:_____AM/PM

**BREAKFAST**    FOODS:    HOW DO I FEEL?

_____:_____AM/PM

**LUNCH**    FOODS:    HOW DO I FEEL?

_____:_____AM/PM

**DINNER**    FOODS:    HOW DO I FEEL?

_____:_____AM/PM

**SNACKS**    FOODS:    HOW DO I FEEL?

**MOOD:**

EXPLAIN WHY:

DID MY ENERGY LEVEL CHANGE?    YES / NO

DID MY BOWELS CHANGE?    YES / NO

WAS MY SKIN AFFECTED?    YES / NO

IS ANYTHING DIFFERENT THAN BEFORE?    YES / NO

HOW DID I FEEL EATING THIS FOOD ITEM?

..................................................................................................
..................................................................................................
..................................................................................................
..................................................................................................

WHAT DID I LEARN ABOUT MYSELF AND MY BODY DURING THIS PROCESS?

..................................................................................................
..................................................................................................
..................................................................................................

WHAT DO I FIND MOST INTERESTING ABOUT THIS PROCESS?

..................................................................................................
..................................................................................................
..................................................................................................
..................................................................................................

WHAT IS MY BIGGEST TAKEAWAY FROM THIS JOURNEY?

..................................................................................................
..................................................................................................
..................................................................................................
..................................................................................................
..................................................................................................
..................................................................................................

WILL I CONTINUE TO EAT THIS FOOD? YES / NO

........ / ........ / ...............

**NEW FOOD ADDITION:** [                    ]

## SLEEP:

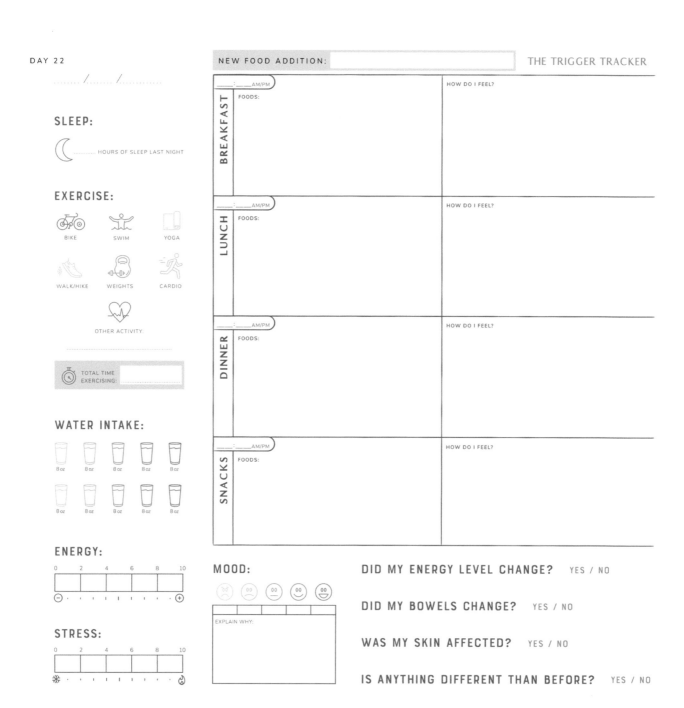

........ HOURS OF SLEEP LAST NIGHT

## EXERCISE:

BIKE    SWIM    YOGA

WALK/HIKE    WEIGHTS    CARDIO

OTHER ACTIVITY:

...........................................

TOTAL TIME
EXERCISING: ...........................

## WATER INTAKE:

8 oz    8 oz    8 oz    8 oz    8 oz

8 oz    8 oz    8 oz    8 oz    8 oz

## ENERGY:

0    2    4    6    8    10

⊖ · · · · · · · · · ⊕

## STRESS:

0    2    4    6    8    10

❉ · · · · · · · · · 🔥

**BREAKFAST**

_____:_____ AM/PM
FOODS:

HOW DO I FEEL?

**LUNCH**

_____:_____ AM/PM
FOODS:

HOW DO I FEEL?

**DINNER**

_____:_____ AM/PM
FOODS:

HOW DO I FEEL?

**SNACKS**

_____:_____ AM/PM
FOODS:

HOW DO I FEEL?

## MOOD:

EXPLAIN WHY:

**DID MY ENERGY LEVEL CHANGE?**   YES / NO

**DID MY BOWELS CHANGE?**   YES / NO

**WAS MY SKIN AFFECTED?**   YES / NO

**IS ANYTHING DIFFERENT THAN BEFORE?**   YES / NO

NEW FOOD ADDITION: _____

........ / ........ / ............

## SLEEP:

( ............. HOURS OF SLEEP LAST NIGHT

## EXERCISE:

BIKE     SWIM     YOGA

WALK/HIKE     WEIGHTS     CARDIO

OTHER ACTIVITY:

........................................

TOTAL TIME
EXERCISING: .......................

## WATER INTAKE:

8 oz     8 oz     8 oz     8 oz     8 oz

8 oz     8 oz     8 oz     8 oz     8 oz

## ENERGY:

| 0 | 2 | 4 | 6 | 8 | 10 |
|---|---|---|---|---|----|

⊖ · · · · · · · · · ⊕

## STRESS:

| 0 | 2 | 4 | 6 | 8 | 10 |
|---|---|---|---|---|----|

✳ · · · · · · · · · ☺

**BREAKFAST**

____:____ AM/PM
FOODS:

HOW DO I FEEL?

**LUNCH**

____:____ AM/PM
FOODS:

HOW DO I FEEL?

**DINNER**

____:____ AM/PM
FOODS:

HOW DO I FEEL?

**SNACKS**

____:____ AM/PM
FOODS:

HOW DO I FEEL?

## MOOD:

EXPLAIN WHY:

DID MY ENERGY LEVEL CHANGE?   YES / NO

DID MY BOWELS CHANGE?   YES / NO

WAS MY SKIN AFFECTED?   YES / NO

IS ANYTHING DIFFERENT THAN BEFORE?   YES / NO

DAY 24

........./........./.............

## SLEEP:

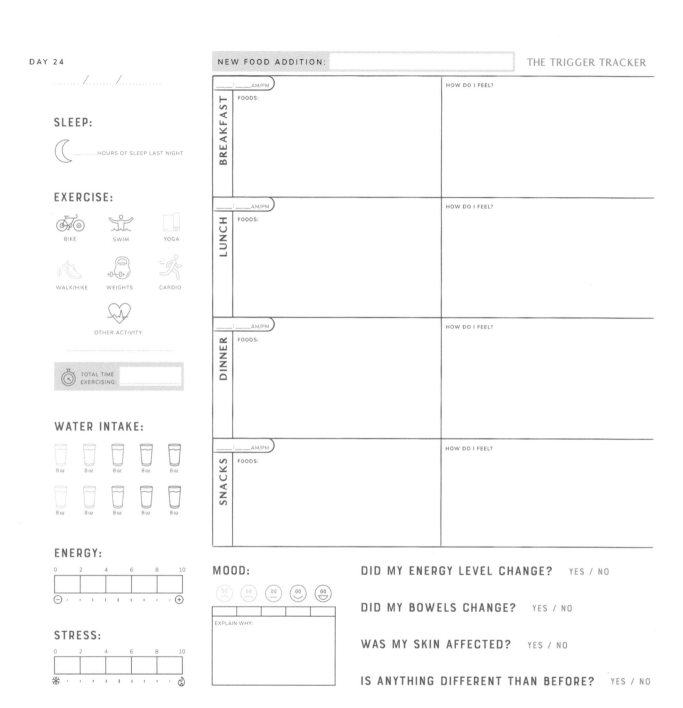

(C ................. HOURS OF SLEEP LAST NIGHT

## EXERCISE:

BIKE    SWIM    YOGA

WALK/HIKE    WEIGHTS    CARDIO

OTHER ACTIVITY:

...................................................

TOTAL TIME
EXERCISING: .........................................

## WATER INTAKE:

8 oz    8 oz    8 oz    8 oz    8 oz

8 oz    8 oz    8 oz    8 oz    8 oz

## ENERGY:

0    2    4    6    8    10

⊖ · · · · · · · · · ⊕

## STRESS:

0    2    4    6    8    10

❇ · · · · · · · · · 🔥

NEW FOOD ADDITION:

**BREAKFAST**
_____:_____ AM/PM
FOODS:
HOW DO I FEEL?

**LUNCH**
_____:_____ AM/PM
FOODS:
HOW DO I FEEL?

**DINNER**
_____:_____ AM/PM
FOODS:
HOW DO I FEEL?

**SNACKS**
_____:_____ AM/PM
FOODS:
HOW DO I FEEL?

## MOOD:

EXPLAIN WHY:

DID MY ENERGY LEVEL CHANGE?    YES / NO

DID MY BOWELS CHANGE?    YES / NO

WAS MY SKIN AFFECTED?    YES / NO

IS ANYTHING DIFFERENT THAN BEFORE?    YES / NO

HOW DID I FEEL EATING THIS FOOD ITEM?

.................................................................................................

.................................................................................................

.................................................................................................

.................................................................................................

WHAT DID I LEARN ABOUT MYSELF AND MY BODY DURING THIS PROCESS?

.................................................................................................

.................................................................................................

.................................................................................................

WHAT DO I FIND MOST INTERESTING ABOUT THIS PROCESS?

.................................................................................................

.................................................................................................

.................................................................................................

.................................................................................................

WHAT IS MY BIGGEST TAKEAWAY FROM THIS JOURNEY?

.................................................................................................

.................................................................................................

.................................................................................................

.................................................................................................

.................................................................................................

.................................................................................................

WILL I CONTINUE TO EAT THIS FOOD?  YES  /  NO

......... / ......... / ...............

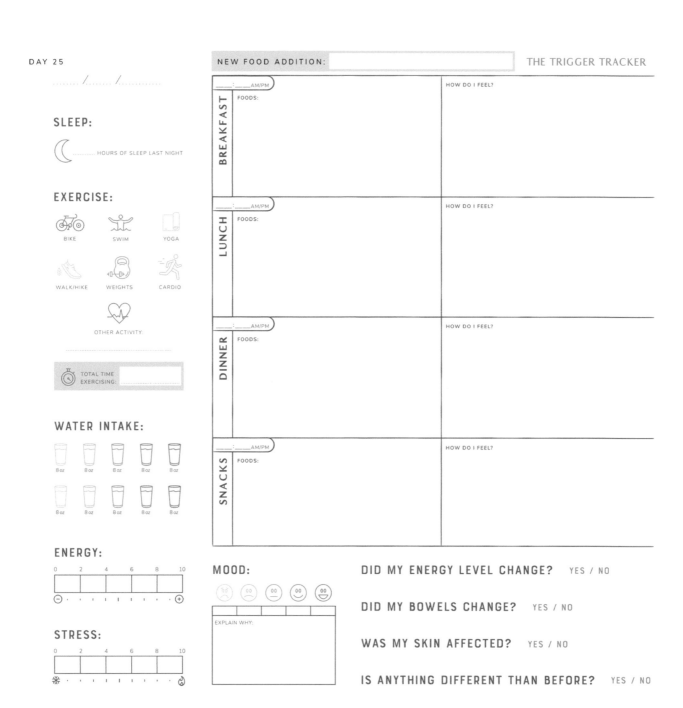

**SLEEP:**

........... HOURS OF SLEEP LAST NIGHT

**EXERCISE:**

BIKE          SWIM          YOGA

WALK/HIKE     WEIGHTS       CARDIO

OTHER ACTIVITY:

.........................................

TOTAL TIME
EXERCISING:

**WATER INTAKE:**

8 oz   8 oz   8 oz   8 oz   8 oz

8 oz   8 oz   8 oz   8 oz   8 oz

**ENERGY:**

0    2    4    6    8    10

⊖                              ⊕

**STRESS:**

0    2    4    6    8    10

❋                              

_____:_____ AM/PM

**BREAKFAST**   FOODS:                     HOW DO I FEEL?

_____:_____ AM/PM

**LUNCH**   FOODS:                     HOW DO I FEEL?

_____:_____ AM/PM

**DINNER**   FOODS:                     HOW DO I FEEL?

_____:_____ AM/PM

**SNACKS**   FOODS:                     HOW DO I FEEL?

**MOOD:**

EXPLAIN WHY:

**DID MY ENERGY LEVEL CHANGE?**   YES / NO

**DID MY BOWELS CHANGE?**   YES / NO

**WAS MY SKIN AFFECTED?**   YES / NO

**IS ANYTHING DIFFERENT THAN BEFORE?**   YES / NO

........../........./..........

## SLEEP:

🌙 ............ HOURS OF SLEEP LAST NIGHT

## EXERCISE:

BIKE          SWIM          YOGA

WALK/HIKE     WEIGHTS       CARDIO

OTHER ACTIVITY.

.......................................

TOTAL TIME
EXERCISING:

## WATER INTAKE:

8 oz   8 oz   8 oz   8 oz   8 oz

8 oz   8 oz   8 oz   8 oz   8 oz

## ENERGY:

| 0 | 2 | 4 | 6 | 8 | 10 |
|---|---|---|---|---|----|

⊖ . . . . . . . . . ⊕

## STRESS:

| 0 | 2 | 4 | 6 | 8 | 10 |
|---|---|---|---|---|----|

❄ . . . . . . . . . ♨

NEW FOOD ADDITION: _____          THE TRIGGER TRACKER

**BREAKFAST**
_____:_____ AM/PM
FOODS:

HOW DO I FEEL?

**LUNCH**
_____:_____ AM/PM
FOODS:

HOW DO I FEEL?

**DINNER**
_____:_____ AM/PM
FOODS:

HOW DO I FEEL?

**SNACKS**
_____:_____ AM/PM
FOODS:

HOW DO I FEEL?

## MOOD:

😞 😟 😐 🙂 😄

EXPLAIN WHY:

DID MY ENERGY LEVEL CHANGE?    YES / NO

DID MY BOWELS CHANGE?    YES / NO

WAS MY SKIN AFFECTED?    YES / NO

IS ANYTHING DIFFERENT THAN BEFORE?    YES / NO

........ / ........ / ...............

**NEW FOOD ADDITION:**

## SLEEP:

............ HOURS OF SLEEP LAST NIGHT

## EXERCISE:

BIKE

SWIM

YOGA

WALK/HIKE

WEIGHTS

CARDIO

OTHER ACTIVITY:

..............................................

TOTAL TIME
EXERCISING: ...............................

## WATER INTAKE:

| 8 oz | 8 oz | 8 oz | 8 oz | 8 oz |
| 8 oz | 8 oz | 8 oz | 8 oz | 8 oz |

**BREAKFAST**

____:____ AM/PM
FOODS:

HOW DO I FEEL?

**LUNCH**

____:____ AM/PM
FOODS:

HOW DO I FEEL?

**DINNER**

____:____ AM/PM
FOODS:

HOW DO I FEEL?

**SNACKS**

____:____ AM/PM
FOODS:

HOW DO I FEEL?

## ENERGY:

0   2   4   6   8   10

⊖ · ı · ı · ı · ı · ı · ⊕

## STRESS:

0   2   4   6   8   10

❉ · ı · ı · ı · ı · ı · 🔥

## MOOD:

EXPLAIN WHY:

**DID MY ENERGY LEVEL CHANGE?**   YES / NO

**DID MY BOWELS CHANGE?**   YES / NO

**WAS MY SKIN AFFECTED?**   YES / NO

**IS ANYTHING DIFFERENT THAN BEFORE?**   YES / NO

HOW DID I FEEL EATING THIS FOOD ITEM?

......................................................................................................

......................................................................................................

......................................................................................................

......................................................................................................

WHAT DID I LEARN ABOUT MYSELF AND MY BODY DURING THIS PROCESS?

......................................................................................................

......................................................................................................

......................................................................................................

WHAT DO I FIND MOST INTERESTING ABOUT THIS PROCESS?

......................................................................................................

......................................................................................................

......................................................................................................

WHAT IS MY BIGGEST TAKEAWAY FROM THIS JOURNEY?

......................................................................................................

......................................................................................................

......................................................................................................

......................................................................................................

......................................................................................................

WILL I CONTINUE TO EAT THIS FOOD?  YES  /  NO

......../......../............

**SLEEP:**

☾ ............ HOURS OF SLEEP LAST NIGHT

**EXERCISE:**

BIKE          SWIM          YOGA

WALK/HIKE     WEIGHTS       CARDIO

OTHER ACTIVITY:

...................................................

TOTAL TIME
EXERCISING: .........................

**WATER INTAKE:**

8 oz  8 oz  8 oz  8 oz  8 oz

8 oz  8 oz  8 oz  8 oz  8 oz

**ENERGY:**

| 0 | 2 | 4 | 6 | 8 | 10 |
|---|---|---|---|---|---|

⊖ · · · · · · · · · ⊕

**STRESS:**

| 0 | 2 | 4 | 6 | 8 | 10 |
|---|---|---|---|---|---|

✳ · · · · · · · · · 🔥

**NEW FOOD ADDITION:** [_____]

**BREAKFAST**

_____:_____ AM/PM
FOODS:

HOW DO I FEEL?

**LUNCH**

_____:_____ AM/PM
FOODS:

HOW DO I FEEL?

**DINNER**

_____:_____ AM/PM
FOODS:

HOW DO I FEEL?

**SNACKS**

_____:_____ AM/PM
FOODS:

HOW DO I FEEL?

**MOOD:**

EXPLAIN WHY:

**DID MY ENERGY LEVEL CHANGE?**   YES / NO

**DID MY BOWELS CHANGE?**   YES / NO

**WAS MY SKIN AFFECTED?**   YES / NO

**IS ANYTHING DIFFERENT THAN BEFORE?**   YES / NO

........../........../.............

**NEW FOOD ADDITION:** _____

## SLEEP:

🌙 ........... HOURS OF SLEEP LAST NIGHT

## EXERCISE:

BIKE          SWIM          YOGA

WALK/HIKE     WEIGHTS       CARDIO

OTHER ACTIVITY:

.......................................

⏱ TOTAL TIME
EXERCISING: _____

## WATER INTAKE:

8 oz  8 oz  8 oz  8 oz  8 oz

8 oz  8 oz  8 oz  8 oz  8 oz

## ENERGY:

0    2    4    6    8    10

⊖ · · · · · · · · · ⊕

## STRESS:

0    2    4    6    8    10

❄ · · · · · · · · · ♨

---

**BREAKFAST**

____:____ AM/PM

FOODS:

HOW DO I FEEL?

**LUNCH**

____:____ AM/PM

FOODS:

HOW DO I FEEL?

**DINNER**

____:____ AM/PM

FOODS:

HOW DO I FEEL?

**SNACKS**

____:____ AM/PM

FOODS:

HOW DO I FEEL?

---

**MOOD:**

EXPLAIN WHY:

**DID MY ENERGY LEVEL CHANGE?**   YES / NO

**DID MY BOWELS CHANGE?**   YES / NO

**WAS MY SKIN AFFECTED?**   YES / NO

**IS ANYTHING DIFFERENT THAN BEFORE?**   YES / NO

......... / ........ / ...............

**SLEEP:**

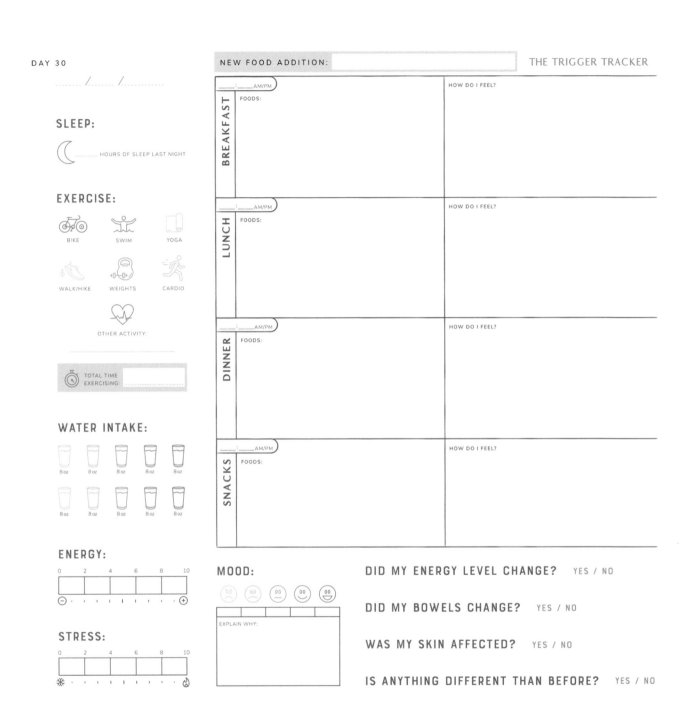

............... HOURS OF SLEEP LAST NIGHT

**EXERCISE:**

BIKE    SWIM    YOGA

WALK/HIKE    WEIGHTS    CARDIO

OTHER ACTIVITY:

...............................................

TOTAL TIME
EXERCISING: ...........................................

**WATER INTAKE:**

8 oz    8 oz    8 oz    8 oz    8 oz

8 oz    8 oz    8 oz    8 oz    8 oz

**ENERGY:**

0    2    4    6    8    10

⊖ · ' ' ' ' ' ' ' · ⊕

**STRESS:**

0    2    4    6    8    10

✳ · ' ' ' ' ' ' ' · 🔥

**BREAKFAST**    _____:_____ AM/PM    HOW DO I FEEL?
FOODS:

**LUNCH**    _____:_____ AM/PM    HOW DO I FEEL?
FOODS:

**DINNER**    _____:_____ AM/PM    HOW DO I FEEL?
FOODS:

**SNACKS**    _____:_____ AM/PM    HOW DO I FEEL?
FOODS:

**MOOD:**

EXPLAIN WHY:

**DID MY ENERGY LEVEL CHANGE?**    YES / NO

**DID MY BOWELS CHANGE?**    YES / NO

**WAS MY SKIN AFFECTED?**    YES / NO

**IS ANYTHING DIFFERENT THAN BEFORE?**    YES / NO

HOW DID I FEEL EATING THIS FOOD ITEM?

...........................................................................................................

...........................................................................................................

...........................................................................................................

...........................................................................................................

WHAT DID I LEARN ABOUT MYSELF AND MY BODY DURING THIS PROCESS?

...........................................................................................................

...........................................................................................................

...........................................................................................................

WHAT DO I FIND MOST INTERESTING ABOUT THIS PROCESS?

...........................................................................................................

...........................................................................................................

...........................................................................................................

...........................................................................................................

WHAT IS MY BIGGEST TAKEAWAY FROM THIS JOURNEY?

...........................................................................................................

...........................................................................................................

...........................................................................................................

...........................................................................................................

...........................................................................................................

WILL I CONTINUE TO EAT THIS FOOD?   YES  /  NO

Printed in the United States
by Baker & Taylor Publisher Services